30.18

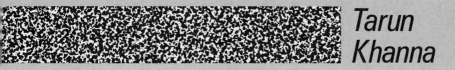

Tarun
Khanna

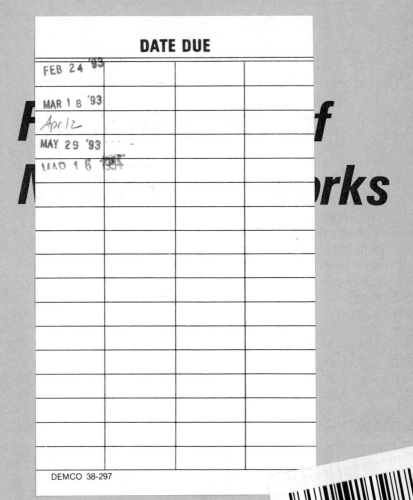

orks

D1023827

▲
▼▼ *Addison-Wesley Publishing Company*

Reading, Massachusetts • Menlo Park, California
New York • Don Mills, Ontario • Wokingham, England
Amsterdam • Bonn • Sydney • Singapore • Tokyo
Madrid • San Juan

This book is in the Addison-Wesley Series in New Horizons in Technology

Library of Congress Cataloging-in-Publication Data

Khanna, Tarun.
  Foundations of neural networks/Tarun Khanna.
    p. cm.
  Includes bibliographical references.
  ISBN 0-201-50036-1
  1. Neural circuitry. 2. Neural computers. I. Title.
QP363.3.K43 1990
006.3—dc20   89-17597
                                                                      CIP

■ *To my family*

Preface

This book was written for the uninitiated, though technically minded, reader. As the title implies, its intended purpose is to serve as an introduction to neural networks. The book captures in print the essence of the evolution of my thought processes over the course of a two-year involvement with neural nets. The book will have served its purpose adequately if an individual with a background similar to mine can peruse the text and arrive at my level of understanding in a period considerably shorter than two years and, perhaps more importantly, with considerably less pain. There has been a tremendous resurgence of interest in neural nets recently. I am one of the individuals who meandered into it from a peripherally related discipline (my formal training is in electrical engineering and computer science) only to find myself immersed in a morass of literature with little to guide me through it. Hence the motivation for this project.

Of my introductory comments above, two things cry out for elaboration. When I speak of my "background," I refer primarily to training in some technical discipline. There is some mathematics in this book. While I have made a conscious effort to keep the math simple and get into details only when it enhances the flow of ideas, I do not believe that this subject can be approached without some basic technical sophistication. Equally important are some nebulous qualities that I would look for in the reader—a predisposition towards studying a subject whose boundaries are by no means clearly defined and an innate curiosity about the interface between relevant modern technology and the ultimate technology of all times, the human brain. Indeed, it is the interdisciplinary nature of the field that attracted me to it in the first place. The study of neural networks owes its origin to fields as diverse as biology, computer science, psychology, and statistics, among others.

The sequence of the chapters will propel the reader from a medley of historical information and basic terminology in Chapter 1 through some key models used in this field in Chapters 2–5 and finally to a discussion of some ways of looking at larger networks in Chapter 6. Yet each chapter can be viewed as a module of sorts and has sufficient references within it to make its relation to the other chapters clear. I have tried, where possible, to go beyond mere descriptions of network models devised by researchers in the field and to examine the motivations underlying the development of those models.

The reader should note that this book does not purport to be a comprehensive reference for the study of neural nets. My aim has been to lay a foundation for further study by unifying the existing literature. Where the lack of time or the scope of the work has prevented me from including something that I felt might have been of some interest to the reader, I have made a mention in the Literature Overview found at the end of each chapter. This section also points out the principal sources for the material on which the chapter is based (bibliographic details can be found at the end of the book). Extended mathematical models, figures, and clearly defined sections of text attributable to a particular publication are referenced within the text of the chapter. I lay no claim to being the originator of any of the concepts, models, or theorems in this book and if, by my error, any acknowledgment is missing or is incorrect, the offended party has my sincerest apologies.

Acknowledgments

I started this project at Princeton with no intention of turning it into a book. Professor Ken Steiglitz at the Department of Computer Science, Princeton University, must be given credit for putting me on the trail of this fascinating field and for subsequently encouraging me to consider publishing what was then a very preliminary report. The comments and suggestions made in recent months by Professor Brad Dickinson at the Department of Electrical Engineering, Princeton University, have been phenomenally helpful. I am indebted to him for essentially upgrading the quality of this project considerably. Additional manuscript reviews that I found beneficial came from Casimir C. "Casey" Klimasauskas, the founder of NeuralWare, Inc., and Dr. Alastair D. McAulay of Wayne State University.

Tom Robbins and his merry team at Addison-Wesley deserve thanks for their patience with a novice. If I had to do this over, I do not think I would make a different choice.

I want to thank Diana for putting up with all the frustrations that have accompanied this project, particularly in its initial stages, and Bhuvnesh, for his incomparable hospitality at Princeton this year. Finally, thanks to my family for their support, and friends in Princeton and elsewhere for their constant encouragement.

Tarun Khanna
Princeton, May 1989

Contents

■ Chapter 6: The Hopfield and Hoppensteadt Models   135

Chapter One

Introduction

■ *1.1 Introduction*

Humans continually process information relevant to "natural" situations (e.g., assimilating a scene or understanding speech) faster than machines. Yet humans are inherently relatively slow and imprecise. This suggests that the computational framework within which machines are being used could probably profit from some revisions on both the architectural and the software levels. Specifically, consider the ability of the human brain to resolve vision and language problems in a few hundred milliseconds. Given the fact that the brain's neural elements have a basic computing speed of a few milliseconds, this implies a processing complexity on the order of a hundred time steps. The best artificial intelligence (AI) programs for comparable tasks are not nearly as general and require millions of computational time steps. The rapid solution of such complex problems is feasible in one of two ways. Information transmission between the computing units may be exceedingly rapid. Unfortunately modern technology has not evolved to the point where the large fan-out seen in the delicately intermeshed structure of the human brain could be imitated on a very large-scale integration (VLSI) chip. Alternatively, we may hypothesize that it may not be necessary to move much information around because the complex structures needed for the problem's solution might be encoded in the neuronal interconnection pattern. It is this latter notion that has given birth to *connectionism*.

As an example, consider the processing involved in understanding a spoken sentence. In order to comprehend the message being communicated, the human brain must not only understand the meaning of the individual words and phrases that comprise the sentence, it must also consider other factors like the context within which the sentence was spoken and the nuance contained in the tone. There are numerous factors that need to be resolved simultaneously before the brain can actually "process" the sentence. Conventional computer systems are not equipped to deal with the vast multitude of mutually interacting factors encountered in such tasks and face the additional problem of requiring that the information they receive be very precisely specified. It would be hard to believe, for instance, that the brain assigns a precise numeric value to the inflexion of voice in a spoken sentence in order to facilitate its processing. Parallel distributed processing (PDP) models (also called neural nets, connectionist models, or neuromorphic systems) propose to address these problems. PDP models are comprised of a large number of simple processing elements called units, each interacting with others via excitatory and inhibitory connections. The large number of units, coupled with the fact that the interconnectedness is primarily local, introduces substantial fault-tolerance. Altering the degree of interconnectedness (i.e., the weight associated with a connection) permits adaptability to new situations.

In theory, it should be possible to form some sort of conventional statistical model that incorporates several factors into making a decision on, for instance, a problem of speech recognition. It is worth mentioning at the outset that there are some important differences between statistical and neural net systems. Just as the parameters of statistical models are derived from training data, so also the neural net "learns" by incorporating past experience into its interconnection patterns. Whereas the statistical model, when confronted by a classification problem, proceeds to serially compute the most likely classification, the neural net performs this computation in parallel and uses the results of its computation to adjust its interconnection patterns. The statistical system parameters determined from historical training data do not change to reflect the new data that can be inferred from the conjunction of the new problem and the system's solution to the problem.

Newell has compiled some historical notes on artificial intelligence and has presented a view of the issues that have existed at various times during the evolution of the field as a series of often concurrently existing dichotomies (e.g., "analog versus digital" or "symbolic versus continuous systems"). In the following few paragraphs a brief outline of these notes attempts to trace, in terms of very broad historical trends, the events leading to the birth of connectionism. We start by postulating that there are three broad classes of systems that may be used as paradigms for the description of intelligent systems—continuous, logic, and symbolic systems. These correspond to the circuit, logic, and program levels in our conventional computers. One of the major historical events relevant to AI in the 1960s was the emergence of two distinct schools of thought along the lines of the continuous and symbolic systems (see Fig. 1.1). These schools gave birth to the cyberneticians (continuous systems) on the one hand and the AI community (symbolic systems) on the other. Beyond the early McCulloch-Pitts efforts to model the neural system, there has been no real effort to use logical systems as the basis for studying intelligent systems. One reason suggested for this is based on the clearly postulated hierarchy between the three levels (i.e., circuits leading to logic levels leading to programs). All that the logic systems could build up to were the program systems. Since program systems were already accounted for by the symbols school, logic systems were rendered redundant. On the other hand, the school concerned with continuous systems did not have to follow this hierarchy because there was always the brain to model.

This continuous/symbolic dichotomy gave rise to and was then re-enforced by other concurrently existing dichotomies. The cyberneticians dealt primarily with pattern recognition and were concerned with developing systems that learned. The AI community, on the other hand, concentrated on problem solving and therefore on creating systems that performed specific tasks demanding intelligence, for example, theorem proving and game-playing. Predictably, each of these groups of tasks was easier to tackle in its specific class of systems. For example, it is easier to tackle a game-playing exercise in a programming system than in a continuous system. Simultaneously, cyberneticians were preoccupied with neurophysiology and the AI community with psychology. While the former connection is easier to understand, the latter arose primarily because it is easier to postulate psychologically meaningful results using programming systems than it is to postulate physiologically meaningful ones. Their preoccupation with neurophysiology led cyberneticians to deal primarily with highly parallel systems. The programming sys-

Figure 1.1 *Parallel strands in the history of artificial intelligence.*

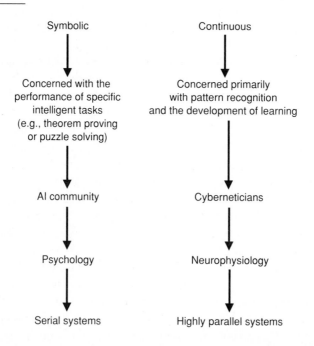

tems employed by the AI community were, on the other hand, inherently serial.

Then, in the 1960s, the AI community became interested in pattern recognition. Until then, this had been strictly the domain of cyberneticians. The AI community, with its use of symbols, was more suited to the construction of scenes than was the pattern-recognition community. With the development of rule-based systems (used for constructing expert systems and analyzing human cognition), there also arose a greater interest in learning among the AI community. Finally, work done in the 1970s on developing algorithms that could perform low-level vision functions introduced a new connection between AI and neuroscience, and this connection initiated the use of highly parallel network structures by the AI community. This new commitment to parallelism should be distinguished from the coarser-grained parallelism employed for some time by the AI community to model an intelligent system as a series of communicating subprocesses, each of which is based on the symbolic paradigm. The finer-grained parallelism resulting from the new connectionist systems communicates more than just significant results between subsystems.

Connectionism may thus be viewed as a marriage of two long-standing schools of thought (see Fig. 1.2). The preceding paragraphs have already introduced the concept of "adaptation" (to new data from which more "learning" may proceed) in neural networks. The *relaxation property* of a network refers to its method of iteratively approaching the best solution to the problem. A detailed discussion of relaxation is best left

Figure 1.2 *Two approaches to artificial intelligence.*

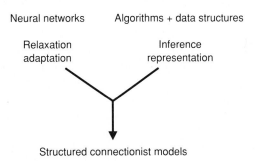

From Feldman, "Computing with Structured Neural Networks," Computer, March 1988. ©1988 IEEE. Reprinted with permission.

until later, for example, in the discussion of the minimal energy concept as a motivation for network dynamics in Chapter 6. The algorithmic/data structures branch of the AI mainstream is concerned with the work being done in structuring conventional AI techniques for conventional serial computers. As already mentioned, one of the premises upon which connectionism is based is that complex constructs necessary for a problem's solution may already be encoded within the interconnection pattern, and, it is the interconnection pattern in a connectionist model that forms the analogue to the algorithm for a conventional serial computer.

It could be argued that any complicated thought process is inherently sequential. For instance, the proof of a theorem in mathematics involves going through a series of logical steps. It is true that the human cognitive process breaks down a complex problem into stages and solves them one at a time; however, PDP models are not concerned with modeling this sequential macrostructure of cognition. Rather, these models focus on the manner in which each of the stages constituting a complex problem is resolved. It is conjectured that the human biological apparatus would be unable to resolve each of these stages in a sequential manner (i.e., there is some parallelism involved). The fact that humans are able to solve problems faster when they can efficiently employ additional constraints and the fact that an entirely sequential process takes longer as additional constraints are incorporated lends credence to such a conjecture. Therefore, a process that is serial on the macro level may have to employ parallel processing to take it, in an efficient manner, from one of its macro states to the next.

Chandrasekaran's (1981) work on natural and social system metaphors for distributed problem solving renders this belief in human parallel computation more plausible. The division of labor among the bees in a hive and the manner in which most modern corporations are organized are two of the examples Chandrasekaran suggests. As mentioned above, incorporation of several constraints can make a thought process exceedingly complicated. Distributing the computation involved among several processors can cut down extensively on memory and time cost. An idea that we will encounter repeatedly throughout this book, and one that consequently cannot be overemphasized, is that of each processor depending primarily on local linkages to do its processing. Adaptation to external changes, a process that all human beings are continually undergoing, is relatively easily done in a system employing distributed processing. For example, a single processor might be replaced with a collection of processors and largely local changes in processor linkages will allow the change in the environment to be effectively dealt with. Distributed processing also allows each processor to be simpler than what it would have to be if it were solving the entire problem. Therefore, replication of processors is possible. One need not be reminded of the billions of neurons in the human brain to realize that replication, to a greater or lesser degree, is indeed a naturally occurring phenomenon. Thus, the modeling of the microstructure of human cognition as a parallel process performed by a distributed architecture, while preserving its sequential macrostructure, is a process that has its analogues in both natural and social systems.

It is important to appreciate that the emergent properties of each distributed architecture represent a particular stage in a sequential thought process. The term *emergent properties* needs some elaboration. Contrary to conventional work done in learning issues in the recent past, PDP models are not constructed to learn by formulating a collection of explicit rules. Rather, the result of the parallel distributed processing should be such that it appears in hindsight as though the model did indeed know those rules. The information required for the architecture to perform the charade of "knowing the rules" is to be contained within the connection strengths between the processors that comprise the architecture. PDP models are concerned with formulating simple, local connection strength modulation mechanisms such that the strengths are always adjusted to reflect changes in the environment. We will examine, primarily in Chapter 2, some of the reasoning underlying distributed architectures and their emergent properties.

The degree to which a distributed architecture is employed in a PDP model varies. PDP models could, in fact, be divided into two classes based upon the extent to which they employ the distributed processing paradigm. Whereas in the local models it is the activity of a single unit that represents the degree of participation of a known conceptual entity, in the distributed models it is a pattern of activity over several units that determines the same degree of participation. Thus, for example, the interactive activation paradigm presented in Chapter 5 is a local PDP model whereas the Hopfield net presented in Chapter 6 is a distributed PDP model.

Smolensky (1986) treats the interesting observation that both the mind and the brain can be studied using PDP models, that is, a PDP model can have either a neural interpretation or a conceptual interpretation or both. Thus a unit in the mathematical world could correspond to a neuron in the brain or a conceptual hypothesis or both. Similarly, the greater the mathematical unit activation, the higher the neuron spiking frequency or the greater the confidence degree in a hypothesis or both.

There is potential for ambiguity when it becomes possible to map a mathematical abstraction into more than one reality. For example, in the case of the Hopfield net there is no apparent conceptual interpretation, but in the case of the model for the interactive activation paradigm we may choose to identify individual neurons with individual words (thus giving the model a local interpretation) or we may choose to give it a distributed neural interpretation. The critical point is that the neural and the conceptual interpretations of a particular mathematical model are entirely independent of each other. It is conjectured that the fact that the same mathematics may be used to describe both the neural and the conceptual levels suggests that PDP modeling might have captured the critical aspects of neural processing.

This book is an attempt to make the vast body of neural-net literature more comprehensible to the uninitiated reader. Rather than merely recount the properties of the several network models devised by researchers in the field, an attempt has been made to examine the motivations behind some of the principal work. Connectionism is, by its very nature, an interdisciplinary field. The motivations behind it are, therefore, often to be found in fields as varied as statistics, psychology, and biology. Some caution is well advised before one is swept away by the exciting possibilities that some of the models appear to promise. The connotation of the brain is very evident in the term *neural networks* and a lot of attention has been paid to the biological aspects of the idea of studying massively parallel realizations of intelligent activity. Computational theory, hardware, and software issues should be accorded equal importance. While switching times of modern-day electronic components are a million times faster than the time that neurons take to change state, our artificial models face severe size constraints. One has only to remember that for conventional chips a fan-out of five is about maximal and that the brain commonly employs much larger fan-out and fan-in to realize that simulating something like a retinal ganglion having more than 10^6 cells is impractical. We have to bear in mind, therefore, that while natural parallel computational solutions have important insights to offer, their practical implementations (with current technologies) will require some modification. Some issues of algorithmic complexity touched upon in Chapter 4 lend credence to this statement.

The ideas and concepts introduced in the remainder of this chapter are presented to help unify the material that appears in subsequent chapters. Much of this book is concerned with PDP models. The section that follows contains a sweeping overview of some of the basic ideas in PDP modeling and of some of the terminology that is an integral part of the vocabulary of a PDP modeler. The concluding part of this introductory chapter provides a chapter by chapter synopsis of the rest of the book.

A few words regarding the manner in which this book deals with references are appropriate here. The bibliography at the end of the book references all publications that were used in the writing of this book. Extended mathematical models, figures, and localised sections of text attributable to a particular publication are referenced within the text. In all other instances, the literature overview section at the end of each chapter discusses the sources from which the primary ideas contained in that chapter were drawn. Where appropriate, additional sources of reference reading are also mentioned, but there has been no attempt to provide an exhaustive list of references. Extensive bibliographies are available elsewhere (e.g., see Klimasauskas (1987)).

■ *1.2 Major Aspects of PDP Models*

Rumelhart (1986a) enumerates the eight major aspects of a parallel distributed processing model as

1. Set of processing units,

2. State of activation,

3. Output function for each unit,

4. Pattern of connectivity,

5. Propagation rule for propagating patterns of activities,

6. Activation rule for combining inputs affecting a unit with its present state to produce an output,

7. Learning rule whereby interconnections can be modified on the basis of experience, and

8. Environment within which the learning system must operate.

Though all of the issues already discussed come up repeatedly in the rest of this book, there are a few concepts that deserve elaboration at this stage. The processing units might represent objects such as features, letters, and the like (which would correspond to what we described earlier as a local PDP model) or abstract elements over which meaningful patterns can be defined (as in a distributed PDP model). The simplest node sums a collection of weighted inputs and passes the result through a nonlinearity. The processing unit is therefore characterized by an internal threshold or offset θ and by the kind of nonlinearity (e.g., hard limiters, threshold logic, or sigmoidal nonlinearities). Figure 1.3 shows a very simple processing unit using a hard-limiting nonlinearity. The nonlinearity here simply seeks to classify the weighted sum of the two inputs as being greater than or less than zero and accordingly assigns the input pattern (i_1, i_2) the value $+1$ or -1 (in this example the offset is presumed to be zero). The relative magnitudes of the weights w_1 and w_2 decide the relative importance of the inputs i_1 and i_2 in determining the final output. Thus, for example, setting w_1 to zero would imply that the outcome of the function merely reflected the sign of the input i_2. The weights have the effect of determining a line in the two-dimensional plane such that all points on one side of the line are distinguished, by the function output, from all those on the other side. Further, a positive value for w_1 would imply that the input i_1 was excitatory to this particular node, whereas a negative value would mean that it was inhibitory. The earliest neurons, of the McCulloch-Pitts kind, were binary threshold devices and a stochastic algorithm involving sudden 0–1 or 1–0 changes of states of neurons at random times was used in the modeling of neuronal systems. As we will see in the discussion of the Hopfield model in Chapter 6, it can be shown that the properties of the original binary model remain intact even when the processing units have a continuous input-output (i/o) relationship.

An interunit interconnection (whose biological analog is a synapse) may be characterized by two features: (1) its nature (i.e., whether it is excitatory or inhibitory) and (2) the degree of influence that the unit from which the interconnection begins has on the incident unit — this is represented by the weight associated with the interconnection. Modification

Figure 1.3 *Processing unit using hard-limiting nonlinearity.*

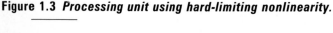
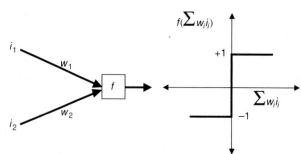

of the interconnections typically implies modification of the associated weights and occurs whenever the neural net learns something in response to new inputs or changes in the environment. Learning strategies are the focus of much of the research in the field and are elaborated to some extent in the rest of this book. At this introductory juncture, however, a cursory description of the forms of some of the rules should suffice.

By far the most common, not only in its original form, but also as a source of many modifications, is the elegant learning rule, due to D.O. Hebb (1949), which suggests that when a cell A repeatedly and persistently participates in firing cell B, then A's efficiency in firing B is increased. The mathematical expression proposed by Sutton (1981) as a widely accepted approximation of this *Hebbian rule* is

$$w_i(t + 1) = w_i(t) + cx_i(t)y(t),$$

where $x_i(t)$ is one of the inputs to the node whose output is $y(t)$ and c is a positive constant determining the rate of learning.

One of the earlier rules proposed for synaptic modifiability was that an afferent (incoming) synapse c_i, initially excitatory, becomes ineffective if and only if the postsynaptic cell fires without presynaptic activity of the cell x_i. This is clearly an inadequate rule as a chance improper stimulus would cause permanent damage to the interconnection.

The Hebbian rule is designed to train the network to function as a pattern associator. Presentation of a stimulus pattern should cause the network to generate another pattern that it has learned to associate with this pattern. Alternatively, presentation of a portion of a pattern should cause the network to generate the complete version of that pattern. This is basically the idea of content addressability and of associative memory and is dealt with in detail in Chapter 2. It may be argued that it is possible to implement addressability using serial computation. For example, one might simply cycle through a list of all possible patterns that an input pattern could possibly be associated with and produce that output which is least dissimilar, but this could easily prove to be quite inefficient. Even the success of more efficient indexing schemes is predicated on the input key being error free. Now, to see how content addressability is implementable with a network of interconnected processors, consider a situation wherein each memory element is connected by mutually excitatory connections with each of the memory units that represent its properties. This would result in content-addressability because the activation of any one or more of its properties (by an input pattern) would cause it to be activated also. Note also that with such a scheme the activation of a unit representing a particular property would cause the simultaneous activation of all memory units that share that property. Since the excitation of a common property could result in a combinatorial explosion of sorts, many of the PDP models include provisions to incorporate lateral inhibition, simply comprised of mutually inhibitory connections between mutually incompatible concepts. We shall see this, for instance, in the discussion of competitive learning in Chapter 5.

The Hebbian rule can be considered as a special case of a generalized learning rule formulated as follows. A synaptic weight increases or decreases in proportion to a reinforcement signal r:

$$w_i(t + 1) = w_i(t) + cr_i(t),$$

where $r_i(t)$ is the reinforcement signal to synapse i at time t, and c is the learning rate. Within this framework the reinforcement signal for the Hebbian rule is given by $r_i(t) = x_i(t)y(t)$.

Learning rules that are essentially connectionistic in character need not imply a locationalistic view of memory. In fact any application of simultaneous, or spatial, correlation can be cast in a form that a Hebbian rule can implement. The temporal subtleties of classical conditioning, however, are not produced by the Hebbian rule even with the use of delays and other modifications. This has led Sutton and Barto, Sutton (1981), to propose their own model, elaborated to some extent in Chapter 2, which provides an interesting development to the conventional models of associative conditioning.

Another example of a learning rule that fits in the general category defined above, is the *Widrow-Hoff rule*. The reinforcement signal is defined as:

$$r_i(t) = [z(t) - y(t)]x_i(t),$$

where

$$y(t) = \sum_{j=1}^{n} w_j(t)x_j(t).$$

This rule causes the weights to converge so that the response is a particular desired real number for each stimulus. If, for example, during the presentation of each stimulus pattern X_α, $\alpha = 1, \ldots, k$, the value to be associated with it is presented as z_α, then after sufficient repetitions of the pairs, the element will respond with z_α when presented with X_α alone. The rule implements an iterative algorithm for computing a solution to a set of linear equations. A solution exists if the stimulus patterns $X_1, \ldots, X_k$ are linearly independent. When Hebbian synapses are employed, perfect recall of Z_α on presentation of X_α is possible only when the stimulus patterns form an orthogonal set. Using the Widrow-Hoff rule, perfect recall occurs even if the stimulus pattern set is only linearly independent. Since nonorthogonal patterns are orthogonalized by the network (of neuronlike elements relying on the Widrow-Hoff rule), this is called *orthogonal learning*. More of this is mentioned in Chapter 2.

The level of activation of the units taken collectively represents the state of the system, and it is convenient to look on the processing carried out by the system as the evolution of this system state. Now, activation of any particular unit induces or hinders the activation of units to which it is connected according to whether the interconnection is excitatory or inhibitory. The notion of activation per se may be viewed in two different ways. First, the activity of a unit indicates its degree of confidence that its associated feature is present or absent, as opposed to merely providing a yes/no answer regarding the presence or absence of a feature. Alternatively, the activity of a unit might suggest the quantity of a feature that is present.

Much work on fuzzy set theory can be related to both these interpretations of activation. As it relates to cognition and neural networks, the basis for the fuzzy set theories depends on what is called the *principle of incompatibility* (i.e., as the complexity of a system increases, our ability to make precise and yet significant statements about its behavior diminishes until a threshold is reached beyond which precision and significance, or relevance, become almost mutually exclusive characteristics). The human brain's ability to summarize, and therefore to approximate, information is essential in view of the plethora of information that has to be synthesized. The key elements of cognition are not numbers, but labels of fuzzy sets (i.e., classes of objects in which the transition from membership to nonmembership is gradual rather than abrupt). This, essentially, is what the notion of "activation" is designed to capture.

The level of activity of a particular unit is provided by an activation function. Williams (1986) introduces the notions of uniform monotonicity and monotonicity-in-context to limit the class of functions that might be regarded as activation functions. Let the set of activation values be in $I = [0, 1]$. Then an activation function is simply $\alpha: I_n \rightarrow I$, when the unit has n inputs and one output. By allowing only the kth coordinate to vary, we define a single-variable section of the function α along the kth coordinate, which is parametrized by the fixed coordinates. Then,

→ α is monotonic-in-context if it is monotonic along all its coordinates (i.e., for each k, all its sections along the kth coordinate are monotonic); and

→ α is uniformly monotonic if it is monotonic along all its coordinates, and for each k, all its sections along the kth coordinate are monotonic in the same sense (i.e., all are nondecreasing or all are nonincreasing).

Clearly, uniform monotonicity implies monotonicity-in-context, but the converse may not be true. The usual sense of excitatory or inhibitory inputs is meaningful exactly when the unit's activation function is uniformly monotonic. Monotonicity-in-context of the activation function may imply an inability to categorize the inputs as solely excitatory or solely inhibitory.

■ 1.3 What Follows . . .

Much of the reason for the attention being paid to neural nets (as opposed, for example, to static statistical classification systems) results from the ability of neural nets to adapt to new environments. It seems reasonable, therefore, to classify them on the basis of their learning strategies. One such classification is based on whether the learning stages are done in the presence of a supervising "teacher" or not. Nets trained under supervision are used as associative memories; those that undergo unsupervised learning are used as vector quantizers or to form clusters. Training is said to be supervised if, during the presentation of an input pattern, the correct class for the input pattern is also specified. Figure 1.4 presents one example of such a classification. The reader need not be concerned with some of the unfamiliar terminology that the figure introduces. The lowest tier of the figure, for instance, lists standard algorithms most similar to the corresponding neural net (in the tier above the lowest). This book is not concerned with the description of these algorithms. We shall, however, make references to the supervised versus the unsupervised learning strategies throughout the book. As it turns out, the difficulty of finding a powerful supervised strategy for learning in networks with hidden layers is a motivation for the development of unsupervised learning strategies. We shall see more of this in Chapter 4.

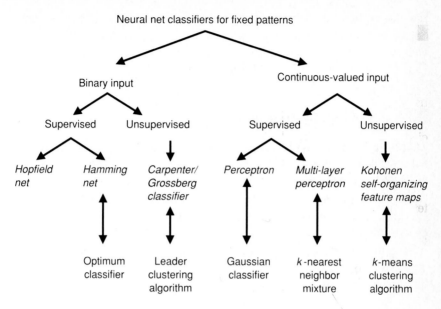

Figure 1.4 *Neural net classifiers for fixed patterns.*

Reprinted with permission from R. Lippman, "An Introduction to Computing with Neural Nets," IEEE ASSP Magazine, April 1987. © 1987 IEEE.

Chapters 2 and 3 are centered around the concept of associative memory. Chapter 2 presents the underlying mathematical basis for the related concepts of associative memory, content-addressing, and the distributed representation of information. Some variants of the Hebbian rule are examined. Chapter 3 focuses on perceptrons and emphasizes the parallel nature of their computational process. Considerable attention is paid to gradient descent techniques and the perceptron convergence procedure is examined. Chapter 4 picks up the theme of gradient descent where Chapter 3 left off and examines learning by back-propagation. Chapter 5 is devoted to the examination of some of the important learning paradigms that have dominated the literature in recent years. Specifically, we present discussions of the competitive learning and the interactive activation paradigms and offer a comparison of the two. It also examines an attempt to stabilize the competitive learning paradigm, the adaptive resonance theory, and then compares this attempt to the learning by back-propagation paradigm introduced in Chapter 4. Finally, Chapter 6 presents two approaches to dealing with large networks— Hopfield nets and the phase-locking approach of Hoppensteadt (1986). The presentation of the Hopfield nets complements the development of the theory of associative memory provided in Chapter 2. Interestingly, both the Hopfield and the Hoppensteadt approaches are unified by an energy surface approach; both types of networks reach stable states by converging to points corresponding to minima on an energy surface.

■ *1. 4 Literature Overview*

Chandrasekaran (1981) has studied naturally occurring instances of distributed computation in information processing. This source provides a brief and simple summary of the advantages and disadvantages of distributed computing and a useful introduction to this notion.

Feldman (1988) is concerned with the design and analysis of specific networks that provide the computational constructs needed to solve hard problems. The paper draws some interesting parallels between the structure of the animal brain and the ability (or inability) of modern technology to imitate nature in this regard.

Hartigan (1975) can be consulted for some standard statistical clustering algorithms.

Lippmann's (1987) introductory paper is an excellent introduction to several basic neural net models. As this book progresses with the description of some of these models, several references will be made to this publication.

McClelland (1986) provides an article that describes the motivations behind PDP models. This article is a chapter in another comprehensive reference in the field of PDP modeling, *(Parallel Distributed Processing, Explorations in the Microstructure of Cognition)*, which will also be referenced on occasion in this book.

Newell's (1983) essay is an interesting starting point for those seeking an introduction to the issues in the AI field. It is not explicitly geared to tracing the motivations surrounding the development of connectionism. Rather, it attempts to dichotomize salient intellectual issues that have held prominence among researchers concerned with artificial intelligence since the 1800s. The enduring impression left by the reading of Newell's article is that created by its emphasis on interdisciplinary issues. We have mentioned in the text of this chapter that connectionism is an interdisciplinary field. This article begins to create an appreciation for the spectrum of issues, and the corresponding spectrum of disciplines, that fuel the long-lasting debates in artificial intelligence.

Smolensky (1986) provides a fascinating mapping from the mathematical PDP models to the neural and conceptual worlds. The interesting observation that the ambiguity in the interpretation of a PDP model arises from the possibility of mapping it in two ways suggests that the very distinct perspectives of the mind and the brain are both informed by the study of PDP models.

Zadeh (1973) postulates that conventional systems analysis techniques, governed in the main by very specific equations, are unsuitable for studying humanistic systems (i.e., nonmechanistic systems). The paper provides an outline of fuzzy set mathematics and the use of linguistic variables where the latter are defined as variables whose values can be described in a natural language.

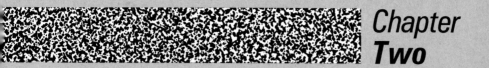

Chapter
Two

Associative Memory

■ *2.1 Introduction*

The ability to get from one internal representation to another, or to infer a complex representation from a portion of it, forms the basis of *associative memory*. Associative memory hinges on the concept of the distributed representation of information. The first part of this chapter is primarily concerned with presenting the theory that motivates these concepts. In the latter half, we present brief discussions of two models that represent a deviation from the view that adaptive changes are a function of co-occurring neuronal events (as exemplified by the Hebbian rule) to a view in which sequential rather than simultaneous events are accorded primary importance.

A conventional computer system has a sequential central processor and a distinct memory unit. To use programs and data stored in memory, it is necessary that the relevant information be directed through the sequential processor. However, in a neural network with a large number of simple interconnected processors, this is no longer true and quick mobilization of information is possible (i.e., the processing time is no longer dominated by the time required to move data/programs to and from memory). Changing connection strengths, or replacing some connections completely by others, causes changes in the contents of memory. Content-addressable memory is hard to achieve in a von Neumann machine (i.e., sequential central processor/passive memory system) because of the latter's accessing of items in memory by using their addresses (and therefore because it is hard to infer the address of a particular item in memory if only a partial description of it is given). For the sake of discussion, assume that an image stored in a conventional computer system has an identifying address and that the presentation of this address to some program generates that particular image as the program output. Now, presentation of a portion of the address will not result in the image being recovered. In contrast, in a neural net employing the associative memory concept, the image is its own address and, in fact, presentation of an approximation of this address will result in the recovery of the actual image as output.

Contemporary memory research focuses more on the mechanisms of encoding and the retention and retrieval of information than on the performance of memory per se. This might be called the adoption of the *memory mechanism paradigm*. In Hinton (1981), memory models are divided into two umbrella categories:

1. *Physical System Models:* These models try to answer the question, How is it possible, using a collection of relatively simple elements

connected to one another, to implement the basic functions of selective associative memory?

2. *Information-Processing Models:* These models conceive of man as an information-processing system executing internal programs for testing, comparing, analyzing, manipulating, and storing information.

This study of associative memory is concerned more with the physical system paradigm. The study of the mechanisms that enable the encoding and subsequent recollection of associations leads to some naturally arising subproblems. It becomes important to identify the neural events that are an integral part of the reading and writing mechanisms, to understand the addressing mechanism used by the nervous system, and to identify the neural elements capable of accumulating memory traces.

■ *2.2 Representation of Information by Collective States*

Because a neural system is an ensemble of a great number of collectively interacting elements, it seems more natural to abandon altogether those physical models of memory in which particular concepts correspond to particular spatial locations (nodes) in the hardware. Instead, we assume that representations of concepts and other pieces of information are stored as collective states of a neural network. Structures of interactions can be made to correspond to structures of knowledge; however, they have no direct physical counterparts in the system—they are realized only through collective effects and are reflected in recall processes. Just as many mathematical or physical entities (e.g., spectral decompositions) can have functional expansions, it is possible to demonstrate that distinct items can be represented as functional components spread all over the memory medium. Therefore, instead of having one unit (neuron) respond if and only if its particular item occurs, each unit responds to many of the possible input items. Provided only one item is presented at a time, it will be represented by the pattern of activity of the internal units even though no individual unit uniquely specifies the input item. Thus a pattern of activity becomes the basic representation of the item. This kind of collective representation might be called *holographic* or *hololalogic*.

Distributed representation of information is not particularly convenient to implement in a conventional von Neumann computer. Rather, it is the efficient manner in which such representations utilize the processing capabilities of neural networks that makes them attractive. From a psychological standpoint, such a representation is rendered plausible by the fact that its strengths and weaknesses match those of the human mind. Each active unit might stand for a microfeature and the connection strengths might represent microinferences between these microfeatures. A stable pattern of activity over all the microfeatures is one that violates the plausible microinferences less than any other neighboring pattern. Modification of the inference rules following the arrival of new information is achieved by modifying the connection strengths. Notice that such an interpretation does not differentiate between actual memory and plausible reconstruction. Such blurring is characteristic of human memory.

Before delving further into this topic of associative memory, the disadvantages of the concept should be noted. The most fundamental problems associated with holographic memory models are cross-talk, communication, invariance, and the inability to capture structure (some of these are elaborated in the next few pages). There is a very real difficulty with having several concepts represented simultaneously in such a system. Hinton (1981) shows that the system with many concepts will be reliable, even for single entries, only if the number of units active for each pattern is proportional to the logarithm of the number of units in the holographic memory. Clearly, as the memory size increases, relatively smaller numbers of units are involved in the representation of any one concept, and this brings us back to localized representation. Another problem is that only one concept can be transmitted at a time between subsystems, if each concept is a pattern on the whole bus. Therefore, for simultaneous communication between a variety of concepts, they must all be represented in disjoint regions. Thus, we are moving further away from the basic idea underlying holographic memory. Finally, consider that a distributed representation is structureless. Given an image of a particular object, for instance, it is not clear how one could generate images of the same object from different perspectives. The way to incorporate structure would be to encode the views from different angles as distinct images. Once again, we violate the tenets of distributed memory.

■ 2.3 Basic Mathematical Model[1]

Hinton (1981) develops the basic linear algebra that underlies the existing conception of associative memory. Suppose we wish to associate patterns of activities f and g, occurring in two distinct sets of n neurons, α

---

[1]Adapted from Hinton, "Models of Information Processing in the Brain," in Hinton (ed.), *Parallel Models of Associative Memory*, Lawrence Erlbaum Associates, 1981. Reprinted with permission.

and β. Suppose further that α and β are completely convergent and divergent (i.e., every neuron in α projects to every neuron in β). Neuron j in α is connected by the $\alpha(i, j)$ weighted synapse to neuron i in β. To bring about the association of f with g, we need to modify synaptic strengths in accordance with the Hebbian rule. Then the change is given by

$$a(i, j) = \eta f(j)g(i).$$

We have an n by n matrix of changes given by

$$\Delta A = \eta g f^T.$$

If f is normalized so that $f.f = 1$ and if $\eta = 1$, then

$$\Delta A = g f^T.$$

If there are m associations (f_1, g_1), (f_2, g_2), $\dots$, (f_m, g_m), then each has an incremental matrix

$$\Delta A_k = g_k f_k^T$$

$$\Delta A = \eta g f^T.$$

If f is normalized so that $f.f = 1$ and if $\eta = 1$, then

$$\Delta A = g f^T.$$

If there are m associations (f_1, g_1), (f_2, g_2), $\dots$, (f_m, g_m), then each has an incremental matrix

$$\Delta A_k = g_k f_k^T.$$

Since there are a finite number of synapses (i.e., n^2) and since, in keeping with the concept of distributed representation, they all store the information collectively, the overall connectivity may be given by

$$A = \sum_k \Delta A_k.$$

Now, if f_k occurs in α, it will cause activity $g = Af_k$ in β:

$$g = Af_k \, \Delta A_k f_k + \sum_{1 \neq k} \Delta A_1 f_k$$

$$= g_k + \sum_{1 \neq k} g_1 (f_1^T f_k)$$

$$= g_k .$$

Therefore, the correct recollection of the pattern associated with the input pattern is dependent on the orthogonality of the patterns f_k. An n-unit linear system with n^2 connections stores n different associations if the input vectors are orthogonal. With nonorthogonality, interference effects, sometimes referred to as *cross-talk*, increase in severity as the number of associations approaches n.

■ 2.4 Associative Recall

Associative recall is a central operation in explaining the functions of distributed memory models. If the memorized data contain proper internal relations, or links, structures of information can be shown to be reflected in the resulting recall processes, that is, without explicitly being represented in memory. In general terms, the basic notion of associative recall is definable as any process by which an input to the memory system, considered as a key, is able to evoke in a highly selective fashion a specific response, associated with that key, at the system output. This implies a specific stimulus-response (S-R) type of mapping in the memory medium, which is able to associate a large number of large-scale activity patterns faithfully and also suppress errors.

The fundamental assumption here is that both the stimulus and response are representable as complex, patterned sets of parallel signals. The mapping is not defined between individual signals but between these activity patterns as a whole, bringing together and interconnecting the various parts of the patterns.

An important note regarding assumptions should be made here. The whole brain is not assumed to be a single uniform network or "matrix," but a complex system consisting of many interacting parts. In the same way as a computer is made of chips of logic circuits, the brain may be composed of a great number of subunits, each one with the properties of a memory matrix.

2.4.1 Mathematical Modeling of Associative Recall[2]

Kohonen (1981) provides another very fundamental analysis of adaptive transformations in distributed associative memory. For the purposes of visualisation, a grid suffices to model the neuronal interconnections. Horizontal lines carry the elements of the stimulus pattern in the form of parallel, scalar-valued signals s_j. The vertical units send out the responses r_i. There is a synaptic connection m_{ij} between every vertical unit i and horizontal line j. For a given set of stimuli s_j to evoke, at the output, another predetermined set of responses r_i, a selective S-R mapping must be encoded into the set of synaptic connections m_{ij}. This encoding is done when signals are mutually conditioned at the connections; the simplest of these conditional couplings is linear mapping. For this conditioning to happen, supervised, nonlinear learning must occur. In our paradigm, the forcing stimuli f_i are needed only when learning or writing into memory occurs; during learning the forcing stimuli have the same signal values as the desired output responses, which thereby become associated with the conditioning stimulus pattern. During recall there is no forcing stimulus present.

Assume that each response signal is a weighted sum of all the stimulus signals and the ith forcing stimulus activity:

$$r_i = \sum_j m_{ij} s_j + f_i,$$

where the weights m_{ij} stand for synaptic conductivities. Assume that the strengths of the m_{ij} are changed during a learning phase by conjunctive forcing—m_{ij} is changed only when both of the signals converging on it are active. If λ, assumed constant, is determined by the plasticity of the connections, we have the following correlation-type learning scheme:

$$\frac{d}{dt} m_{ij} = \lambda f_i s_j.$$

At any instant, there is a stimulus pattern $s = (s_1, \ldots, s_m)$, a forcing stimulus pattern $f = (f_1, \ldots, f_n)$, and a response pattern $r = (r_1, \ldots, r_n)$.

---

[2]Math in Section 2.4.1 from Kohonen, "Distributed Associative Memory," in Hinton (ed.), *Parallel Models of Associative Memory*, Lawrence Erlbaum Associates, 1981. Reprinted with permission.

(All patterns are parallel signals.) Then the vector forms of the above equations are

$$r = Ms + f$$

$$\frac{d}{dt}M = \lambda fs^T.$$

Assume that there are p stimulus vectors and p corresponding forcing vectors (with the superscript being used to distinguish between them). Also assume that $m_{ij} = 0$ initially. Then from the instant $t = 0$ onward, the first pair of stimulus and forcing stimulus vectors $(s^{(1)}, f^{(1)})$ appears at the network inputs and stays there for time t. Then matrix M develops into

$$M(t) = \lambda t f^{(1)} s^{(1)T}.$$

If each of the p pairs appears at the input for $t = 1/\lambda$ time, then M takes the n by m cross-correlation matrix form

$$M = \sum_{i=1}^{p} f^{(i)} s^{(i)T}.$$

Once outside the learning phase, the response is defined without the forcing stimulus (i.e., $r = Ms$). If we assume orthogonality of the key vectors s, then, in much the same way as the analysis carried out above, we can show that presentation of a stimulus s_j causes the response to exactly equal the associated forcing stimulus f_j. Therefore, in a concrete example, $f^{(i)}$ could represent the classification of stimulus $s^{(i)}$ in which case the classification of $s^{(i)}$ would take place very simply by analyzing the response obtained when it was used as the stimulus pattern. In this case, since the maximum number of orthogonal stimulus vectors is m, this is also the maximum number of stimulus-response pairs that can be stored while simultaneously preserving *optimal* recall.

Interestingly, the strong condition of orthogonality is not required to get perfect recall. It is sufficient that the $s^{(i)}$ be linearly independent. Then in fact the correlation matrix is given by

$$M = F(S^T S)^{-1} S^T,$$

where

$$F = (f^{(1)}, \ldots, f^{(p)}) \qquad \text{and}$$

$$S = (s^{(1)}, \ldots, s^{(p)}).$$

If the stimulus vectors $s^{(j)}$ are not linearly independent, the best fit solution in the least-squares sense is given by

$$\hat{M} = FS^+,$$

where

$$S^+ = \text{pseudoinverse of } S.$$

Note: $S^+ = S$ if $s^{(j)}$ are linearly independent.

If $F = S$, then the nontrivial solution to M is given by FF^+ and is called the *orthogonal projection operator*. The p n-dimensional vectors, $f^{(1)}, \ldots, f^{(p)}$, span a linear subspace L in n dimensions. Any n-dimensional vector f can be decomposed into

$$f = \hat{f} + \tilde{f}$$

where

$\hat{f} = FF^+f$ and is the best linear combination of the $f^{(j)}$ in least square terms (*optimal autoassociative recollection* relative to the $f^{(j)}$) and
$\tilde{f}$ = residual.

If the $f^{(j)}$ are orthonormal, then M takes the autocorrelation matrix form

$$M = FF^T = \sum_{i=1}^{p} f^{(i)}f^{(i)T}.$$

Then for any pattern vector f,

$$\hat{f} = Mf = \sum_{i=1}^{p} (f^{(i)T}f)f^{(i)} \qquad \text{and}$$

$$\tilde{f} = f - \hat{f}.$$

Here the optimal autoassociative recollection is clearly expressed as a linear combination of the stored vectors, and the coefficients of the expansion are the inner products of the stored vectors with the new vector f.

Even when the stored vectors are nonorthogonal, there exists a relationship between FF^+ and FF^T, given by

$$FF^+ = \alpha \sum_{k=0}^{\infty} FF^T (I - \alpha FF^T)^k.$$

Since the αFF^T term appears as the 0th degree term in the expansion of the right-hand side of the equation, we may regard the autocorrelation matrix (FF^T) as a 0th degree approximation of the optimal mapping.

2.4.2 The Novelty Component Approach[3]

In the realm of statistics and regression analysis, there would be a negative connotation attached to the residual vector and the object would be to minimize it. Kohonen (1981), however, has pointed out that the residual represents that part of the input vector f that could not be explained by the stored pattern list $f^{(j)}$. In that sense, the residual is the *novelty component*. Note that the residual is the result of a projection by matrix P such that

$$\tilde{f} = f - FF^+f$$

$$= (I - FF^+)f$$

$$= Pf.$$

Note that P projects f onto a subspace that is orthogonal to that spanned by the $f^{(j)}$. We might say that the residual vector represents the result of P's filtering out of novel information that is not associated with the earlier stored vectors.

---

[3]Math in Section 2.4.2 from Kohonen, "Distributed Associative Memory," in Hinton (ed.), *Parallel Models of Associative Memory*, Lawrence Erlbaum Associates, 1981. Reprinted with permission.

2.4.3 A Stochastic Approach to Recall in Large-Scale Operations[4]

Kohonen (1972) provides an analysis of what happens to the above theory when the cross-correlation matrix becomes too large. First, let us picture the model as follows. The input field is composed of the key and the data fields. All input receptors receive a set of simultaneous input signals. Key field and data field signals are denoted respectively by the vectors $q^{(p)}$ and $x^{(p)}$, where the superscript (p) refers to a particular pattern. The associator, or memory element, field has elements labeled by (i, j) corresponding to the ith element of the key field and the jth element of the data field to which the associator is connected. A *complete correlation matrix memory* (CCMM) is one that has connections for all possible pairs (i, j) and only one of a type. An *incomplete correlation matrix memory* (ICMM) has its pairs either selected randomly or generated randomly.

In a CCMM, the associator field is described by the matrix

$$M_{xq} = c \sum_p x^{(p)} q^{(p)^T}.$$

As before, $\hat{x}^{(r)} = M_{xq} q^{(r)}$ is used to recall data, and we can go through the same analysis to demonstrate that perfect recall results from orthogonality of the q vectors. Kohonen (1972) shows that the relative cross-talk level, resulting from nonorthogonality of the key (i.e., q) vectors, for a particular datum is given by

$$L^{(p, r)} = \frac{q^{(p)^T} q^{(r)}}{\|q^{(r)}\|^2}$$

and provides a measure of selectivity.

The analysis for one case of ICMM, *a stochastically sampled correlation matrix,* is as follows. The purpose is to analyze what sort of "noise" or statistical error is introduced when such a correlation matrix is used. When the dimensions of the key and data vectors are increased, the number of matrix entries (mn) grow impractically large. The approach hinges on defining sampling coefficients s_{ij} that take the value 1 at all sampled elements and 0 otherwise. The sampled matrix is

$$(M_{xq})_{ji} = c \sum_p s_{ij} q_i^{(p)} x_j^{(p)}.$$

[4]Math in Section 2.4.3 from Kohonen, "Correlation Matrix Memories, *IEEE Transactions on Computers,* C = 21, No. 4, April 1972. © 1972 IEEE. Reprinted with permission.

The recalled pattern is

$$\hat{x}_j^{(r)} = c \sum_p \sum_{i=1}^m s_{ij} q_i^{(p)} x_j^{(p)}$$

$$= c \left[\sum_{i=1}^m s_{ij} (q_i^{(r)})^2 \right] x_j^{(r)} + c \sum_{p \neq r} \sum_{i=1}^m s_{ij} q_i^{(p)} q_i^{(r)} x_j^{(p)}$$

$$= K_j^{(r)} x_j^{(r)} + \sum_{p \neq r} K_j^{(p,r)} x_j^{(p)}.$$

Here gain factors $K_j(r)$ and $K_j(p, r)$ are stochastic variables. The probability for the stochastic variable s_{ij} being 1 is given by

$$w = \frac{s}{mn},$$

where

s = number of sampled matrix elements,
m = number of components in q, the key vector, and
n = number of components in x, the data vector.

The large size of the data vector (we only use ICMM when the matrix size is large) validates the assumption of a binomial distribution for s_{ij}. Then,

$$E(s_{ij}) = w \qquad \text{and} \qquad \text{var}(s_{ij}) = w(1 - w).$$

Also

$$E(K_j^{(r)}) = cw \sum_{i=1}^m (q_i^{(r)})^2$$

$$\text{var}(K_j^{(r)}) = c^2 w(1 - w) \sum_{i=1}^m (q_i^{(r)})^4.$$

The relative standard deviation due to the searched pattern only is

$$\frac{\sqrt{\text{var}(K_j^{(r)})}}{E(K_j^{(r)})} = \sqrt{\frac{1 - w}{w}} \frac{\sqrt{\sum_{i=1}^m (q_i^{(r)})^4}}{\sum_{i=1}^m (q_i^{(r)})^2}.$$

This term defines the fidelity of recall of a stored pattern. The cross-talk, which was mentioned earlier as an inherent failing of distributed representation, from another pattern p is characterised by the following expressions:

$$E(K_j^{(p,r)}) = cw \sum_{i=1}^{m} q_i^{(p)} q_i^{(r)}$$

$$\text{var}(K_j^{(p,r)}) = c^2 w(1-w) \sum_{i=1}^{m} (q_i^{(p)} q_i^{(r)})^2.$$

Combining this result with the earlier expression for the recalled pattern, we can get an expression for the cross-talk experienced during the recall of pattern r due to all patterns p:

$$\frac{\sqrt{\text{var}(\hat{x}_j^{(r)})}}{E(\hat{x}_j^{(r)})} = \sqrt{\frac{1-w}{w}} \frac{\sqrt{\sum_{i=1}^{m} \left(\sum_p q_i^{(p)} q_i^{(r)} x_j^{(p)} \right)^2}}{\sum_p \sum_{i=1}^{m} q_i^{(p)} q_i^{(r)} x_j^{(p)}}.$$

It is reasonable that this expression approaches 0 as w approaches 1 because this means that we are using a CCMM (i.e., $s = mn$).

■ 2.5 Memory as an Adaptive Filter

The filtering approach evident in the novelty-component interpretation has also been adopted by Kohonen (1977). Memory is regarded as an *adaptive filter* implemented by a neural network. The resulting model can be looked on as a dynamic version of that described by the preceding equations. The adaptive filter model demonstrates how old outputs to previous stimulus-response pairs (which had influenced the synaptic strengths, earlier referred to as m_{ij}) influence the responses to new stimuli. *Writing* comes about when each input pattern produces *adaptive* changes in the neuronal interconnections. *Reading* is the transformation of the input signals in the network. No addressing problem (a characteristic of associative memory) exists since memory traces are spatially distributed and superimposed throughout the network. For such a filter model to make sense, it must have the following features:

1. Cell population is organized in a great number of elementary functional units that form the basic linkages between input and output signals.

2. Associative memory is implemented by modifiable interconnections.

3. Number of interconnections are much greater than the number of functional units.

2.5.1 Biological Basis for Model

It is suggested that the strong vertical connectivity of the cerebral neocortical tissue, to a great extent due to the shape of the pyramidal cells that constitute the principal neurons in the region and to the vertical orientation of the afferent neurons, has the above properties to a desirable extent. Specifically, the vertical cortical columns could be the functional units spoken of in feature 1. The biological evidence is presented in the ensuing discussion in order to provide support for the mathematical aspects of the model and is not intended as a complete discussion of the mammalian cortex. The actual formulation of the computing model of the cortical associative network involves several steps:

1. Structural assumptions,

2. Approximation for the transfer function of the network,

3. Law of synaptic modifiability, and

4. Perturbation approximation of the adaptive effects.

The model also draws substantial evidence from lateral inhibition as a means of preprocessing the afferent patterns and thereby producing an increase in the memory capacity and the selectivity of the neuronal network. As a biological analog, an excitatory signal in the cortex is, as a rule, surrounded by an inhibitory penumbra.

Columnar Organization of the Cortex. Mammalian neocortical tissue is functionally organized in macroscopic units called columns. Cells within a column respond similarly to external stimuli with a particular attribute. Every column has three types of input:

1. Specific afferent axons, which are the principle inputs of external signals to the column (this corresponds to the view of cortical organization that suggests that every column consists of an elementary linkage between the input and output signals);

2. Activity-controlling, nonspecific afferent axons originating in different parts of the brain; and

3. Subcortical association fibres, which interconnect columns in the lateral direction (note that the inclusion of lateral inhibition in the Kohonen (1977) model is of central importance in the achievement of large memory capacity).

The model's basic operating unit is an input-output element (e.g., a single principal cell of the pyramidal type). These elements form a laminar two-dimensional layer in which spatial activity patterns may be thought to occur. A strong connectivity is assumed between the inputs and outputs in a one-to-one fashion (reference the vertically oriented neocortical texture). The input/output units are also connected laterally in two ways: short-range connectivities (intracortical connections primarily responsible for lateral inhibition) and long-range connectivities (these connections, assumed to exist between all input/output pairs in the simulated area, are primarily thought to be responsible for the associative recall function by which missing parts of patterns are reconstructed).

Transfer Function of a Cortical Neural Network. The Kohonen (1977) theory's signal transmission properties are described by the linearized frequency transfer function. In reality, nonlinear differential equations describe neuron triggering dynamics. However, the neuron triggering frequency, averaged over a short time span, relates to the presynaptic impulse frequencies in a way that can be approximated by a linear function. This implies that during the period of being active the neurons' output frequency changes are related linearly to the input frequency changes.

The linearized theory assumes that a functional unit (e.g., a column) modulates the activity of another unit in proportion to its own activity, and that a nonspecific background activity is present. Therefore, every local activity depends on a large number of other local activities:

$$\eta_i = \beta_i \xi_i + \sum_j \mu_{ij} \eta_j + \eta_b',$$

where

ξ_i = input spike frequency,
η_i = output spike frequency,
β_i = direct connection between input and output,
μ_{ij} = long-range connectivity from unit j onto unit i, and
η_b' = defines background activity.

Synaptic Modifiability. Memory traces are identifiable most directly with changes in synaptic connectivities between neuronal pairs. The number of synapses in the cerebral cortex alone (10^{13} to 10^{14}) is sufficiently large to encode every lifetime experience. *Stent's law of plasticity* (Stent 1973) is a modification of the popular Hebbian principle and can be summarised as follows. The efficacy change of a synapse is proportional to the postsynaptic triggering activity, which is either zero or positive; in the first linearized approximation, the changes are assumed to be proportional to the difference between the presynaptic activity and some equilibrium value, at which increasing and decreasing effects attain an approximate balance.

2.5.2 Mathematical Model[5]

Changes in the β_i or the μ_{ij} can be used to demonstrate various memory effects and interesting information processing functions (e.g., feature sensitive detectors). Since changes in the μ_{ij} are sufficient to demonstrate those effects central to selective distributed memory operation, we assume β_i constant with time. The law of synaptic modifiability is similar to the Hebbian principle except for the background activity term:

$$\frac{d\mu_{ij}}{dt} = \alpha\eta_i(\eta_j - \eta_b),$$

where

$$\alpha = \text{synaptic plasticity and}$$
$$\eta_b = \text{average background activity.}$$

If the $\beta_i\xi_i$ term is replaced by the effective input excitation of unit $i\xi_i'$, if the excitations are regarded as spatial patterns $\{\xi_i't_k)\}$, and if the input patterns for $k = 1, 2, \ldots, m$ are switched on for time Δt, then the stepwise solution to the law of synaptic modifiability is

$$\mu_{ij}(t) = \alpha\Delta t \sum_{k=1}^{m} \eta_i(t_k)[\eta_j(t_k) - \eta_b] + \mu_{ij}(0) \qquad t > t_k.$$

Then the output spike frequencies are given by

$$\eta_i(t) = \xi_i'(t) + \alpha\Delta t \sum_j \sum_k \eta_i(t_k)[\eta_j(t_k) - \eta_b]\eta_j(t) + \sum_j \mu_{ij}(0)\eta_j(t) + \eta_b'$$

[5]Math in Section 2.5.2 reprinted with permission from *Neuroscience*, 2, Kohonen, "A Principle of Neural Associative Memory." Copyright © 1977 Pergamon Press plc.

and are seen to be modified by adaptive effects that earlier signals caused in the network. The last equation describes the reading of information from memory. The changes in the output that result as a result of modifications in the network are explainable by the *principle of virtual images*. This basically states that there is a component to the new output that is attributable to memory recollections. Therefore,

$$\eta_i(t) = \xi_i'(t) + \hat{\xi}_i'(t) + \sum_j \mu_{ij}(0)\eta_j(t) + \eta_b',$$

where

$$\hat{\xi}_i'(t) = \text{virtual recollections of information from memory,}$$

and

$$\hat{\xi}_i'(t) = \alpha \Delta t \sum_j \sum_k \eta_j(t)[\eta_j(t_k) - \eta_b]\eta_i(t_k)$$

$$= \sum_k \gamma_i(t, t_k)\eta_i(t_k),$$

that is, these recollections are linear mixtures of old outputs $\eta_i(t_k)$ with weighting coefficients

$$\gamma_i(t, t_k) = \alpha \Delta t \sum_j \eta_j(t)[\eta_j(t_k) - \eta_b],$$

which depend on the similarity of the present outputs $\eta_j(t)$ to the earlier ones.

■ 2.6 The Sutton-Barto Model

Neural network models designed to explore the behavioral possibilities of modifiable structures typically employ a pre- and postsynaptic correlation rule for altering connectivities, which is essentially a mathematical representation of Hebb's postulate. Sutton and Barto, Sutton (1981), take the view that classical conditioning involves an interplay between expectations and stimulus patterns that is too complex to incorporate into a simple correlation rule such as Hebb's. They suggest that the reason for the success of the Hebbian rule is that it provides a simple explanation of stimulus substitution theory. The essence of this theory is precisely what its name implies. Let us, for explanatory purposes, say that stimulus A elicits response R_A. Now, if every presentation of A is associated with the presentation of another stimulus B, then over time, presentation of stimulus B alone also elicits a response similar to R_A. The substitution of stimulus B for stimulus A is said to have occurred. Here, A is the conditioned stimulus (CS) that causes the conditioned response (CR). B is the unconditioned stimulus (UCS) that eventually elicits an unconditioned response (UCR) similar to the CR. Now, consider a threshold element that fires whenever one of its pathways has an input. If another pathway also happens to be have an input when this firing occurs, then it will, by the Hebbian rule, have its weight strengthened. After a while, an input along this second pathway alone will be enough to cause firing. In this fashion, the Hebbian rule is able to account for stimulus substitution.

One of the problems that Sutton and Barto have with this approach is that it allows for the occurence of stimulus substitution only when the conditioned and unconditioned stimuli are presented simultaneously. This is in contrast to empirical data, which suggests that simultaneous presentation of the stimuli results in poor conditioning. Substitution occurs effectively when the CS precedes the UCS. Now the Hebbian rule has no means of accommodating such a temporal relationship. There are further temporal subtleties, such as the time lag between the CR and the CS, that the Hebbian rule is not equipped to deal with. In some sense it is appropriate to say that the predictive aspect of classical conditioning has been largely overlooked by conventional Hebbian rule-based models and it is this deficiency that the Sutton-Barto model seeks to address. The adaptive element presented learns to increase its response rate in anticipation of increased stimulation, producing a conditioned response before the occurence of the unconditioned stimulus. Further, the adaptive element is not constrained by the early perspection of neurons essentially switching elements devoid of much internal processing power. While quite complex computational power is attributed to individual adaptive elements, no attempt is made to suggest that all the mechanisms must reside in each element. In particular, an adaptive element may not correspond to a neuron.

The mathematical formulation of the Sutton-Barto model is as follows. In addition to the stimulus signals x_i, $i = 1, \ldots, n$, and the output signal y, this model requires the use of several other variables. First, for each stimulus signal x_i, we require a separate stimulus trace ξ_i. The occurence of CS_i at time t, indicated by $x_i(t) = 1$, initiates a prolonged trace given by nonzero values of a separate variable ξ_i for some period of time after t. This is accomplished by letting $\xi_i(t)$ be a weighted average of the values of x_i for some time period preceding t. Similarly, we require a trace of the output y. Let $\psi(t)$ denote a weighted average of the values of the variable y over some time interval preceding t. Then we have

$$\xi_i(t + 1) = \alpha\xi_i(t) + x_i(t)$$

and

$$\psi(t + 1) = \beta\psi(t) + (1 - \beta)y(t),$$

where

$$0 \leqq \alpha, \qquad \beta < 1.$$

The values of the associative strengths are given by

$$w_i(t + 1) = w_i(t) + c[y(t) - \psi(t)]\xi_i(t),$$

where c is a positive constant determining the rate of learning.

   The interpretation of the Sutton-Barto model is as follows. Activity on any input pathway $i, i = 1, \ldots, n$, possibly causes an immediate change in the element output y but also causes the connection from that pathway to become "tagged" by the stimulus trace ξ_i as being eligible for modification for a certain period of time (the duration of the trace ξ_i). A connection is modified only if it is eligible and the current value of y differs from the trace ψ of y. The effectiveness of the reinforcement for the conditioning process depends on the difference $y(t) - \psi(t)$, which determines how the eligible connections actually change. The notion of periods of eligibility was borrowed from the neural hypothesis that the temporal characteristics of conditioning, both classical and instrumental, can be produced if one set of conditions makes synapses eligible for modification of their transmission efficacies, but actual modifications occur due to other influences during periods of eligibility. This differs from related theories in that eligibility is seen as being indicated in some way completely separate from electrical activity. Therefore, in this model, prolonged presynaptic activation, for instance, would not make a pathway modifiable. Rather, some mechanism that does not participate directly in the electrical signalling of the cell, such as a transient increase in the concentration of a particular chemical, would determine eligibility.

   Whereas the Hebbian rule detects correlations between input and output signals, this rule detects correlations between traces (i.e., that denoted above by the ξ signals) of input stimuli and changes of output.

The importance of the Sutton-Barto model can be seen from the following. Using the framework for the reinforcement signal introduced in Chapter 1, we have

$$r_i(t) = [\,y(t) - \psi(t)]\xi_i(t)\,.$$

The teacher input, $z(t)$ has been replaced by $y(t)$. This eliminates the requirement that reinforcement be provided only by a fixed reinforcing pathway (where the fixed pathway would be the one used by the teaching input during the supervised learning phase). Since $y(t)$ can be effected by activity on any input pathway, any input signal can bring about changes in the efficacies of other pathways. This permits the adaptive element to extract predictive relationships among its inputs in the same way that a Hebbian element extracts simultaneous associations. Essentially, the need for a distinct channel for reinforcing signals has been eliminated by providing a distinct time (with respect to a conditioned stimulus) for reinforcement.

◾ 2.7 The Heterostat

Klopf (1982), in proposing a theory primarily of intelligent adaptive behavior, provides a broader framework on adaptive systems and places the Hebbian model and the Sutton-Barto model within this framework. Broadly speaking, the two types of connectionist neural models that have been employed in studying adaptive networks are the association and the reinforcement models. The latter is subdivided into the restricted reinforcement models, (of which the Sutton-Barto model is one) and the generalized reinforcement model (of which Klopf's heterostat is one). Before involving ourselves in a discussion of what distinguishes these models from one another, we will examine the heterostat in greater detail.

A salient motivation for Klopf's work appears to be the similarity that he perceives between social and neural systems. Briefly, both systems are constituted of building units—people and neurons. In both cases, these units exhibit substantial convergence/divergence in their interconnection/interaction patterns. Both are adaptive systems, possessing the ability to learn from experience. In both cases, there is redundancy in the interconnection pattern, which permits recovery from damage to individual unit(s) and is a measure of the systems' plasticity. The primary questions concern the nature and location of the mechanisms that allow the systems to be adaptive. The belief that units in a social system form their network connections based on local circumstances (i.e., the adaptive mechanism is localised) spawns the belief that neurons might carry out a similar process in the brain.

Just as people are pleasure-maximizers, so neurons might possess the same hedonistic characteristic. Hedonism implies pleasurable and painful states; for the neuron these are the states of depolarization (pleasure) and hyperpolarization (pain). The mechanistic interpretation of the resulting implication, that a neuron will seek to obtain excitation and to avoid inhibition, is based on B. F. Skinner's theory of operant conditioning as applied to the neuron instead of to a whole organism. If a neuron experiences further depolarization within a few hundred milliseconds of firing, it strengthens the excitatory synapses that caused it to fire; if correspondingly, it experiences further hyperpolarization, those inhibitory synapses that were active at the time of firing are strengthened. Synaptic strength, therefore, encodes a causal relation, providing predictive information concerning the consequences for the neuron if it fires when the synapse is active. Over time, the neuron behaves as an excitation-maximizer and an inhibition-minimizer.

Continuing his social analogy, Klopf points out that the Industrial Revolution taught us about non–goal-seeking systems with non–goal-seeking components. The cybernetic revolution that has taught us the importance of information (and of feedback mechanisms) deals with goal-seeking systems with non–goal-seeking components—called, say, *control systems*. Here, we may regard a goal-seeking system as one that utilizes feedback information to move toward, or to maintain, a particular system state that is the goal. Correspondingly, a non–goal-seeking system is an open-loop system. An *adaptive system* modifies its structure as a function of experience so as to improve relative to some criterion. An *adaptive network* is an adaptive system (with relatively simple units) functioning in a decentralized, highly parallel fashion.

The brain, in as much as it possesses goal-seeking and adaptive characteristics, is definitely a control system. The question is whether we can go further and credit individual neuronal elements in the brain as being goal-seeking also. Klopf argues that modern scientists are unwilling to think of neurons as goal-seeking not only because they have been conditioned by the Industrial Revolution into thinking of non–goal-seeking components but also because the idea of something as small as a neuron possessing the ability and motivation to progress toward a predefined goal is hard to fathom. The non–goal-seeking neuronal nature would imply that the intelligence of the brain was an emergent phenomenon. Klopf maintains that such a view does not lead to an understanding of intelligence because particular kinds of local feedback mechanisms that have been absent from most brain models may be crucial to the emergence of intelligence. Intelligence can be understood only after the assumption that the single neuron is a goal-seeking system in its own right is made.

There are two important points regarding goal-seeking at a neuronal level. First, goal-seeking does not go any further, that is, we assume that the smallest entity that exhibits this property is the cell (neuron). Atoms and molecules are not goal-seeking. Second, the goal being sought has to do with neuronal inputs, not outputs. The single neuron does not have as its goal the act of firing, but rather wants simply to obtain excitation and avoid inhibition. Outputs are not an end in themselves, rather they are a means to an end. They must be manipulated to control inputs.

There is also an important point to be made regarding goal-seeking at the level of the brain. In addition to assuming that basic components are non–goal-seeking, it has also been assumed that the brain seeks to achieve homeostasis—the condition of a system in which a set of "essential variables" has assumed steady-state values compatible with the system's continued ability to function. (Here "essential variables" are those that are required for survival and are dynamically intertwined with each other.) Klopf argues that the latter assumption is misleading. The amount of homeostatic behavior in an organism decreases as the intelligence of the organism increases. In the case of humans, who very often display nonhomeostatic behavior, homeostasis can be thought of as the goal of the autonomic nervous system, but not of the somatic nervous system. The somatic nervous system seeks more to maximize rather than to achieve a steady-state condition. Specifically, the somatic nervous system strives to maximize the difference between the amounts of reward and punishment obtained by it. Therefore, intelligence in complex systems is a concomitant of a striving for a maximal condition termed *heterostasis.*

A clarification of the relative importance of heterostasis and homeostasis is in order. The latter is secondary in importance, but is nonetheless required for survival. In contrast, maintaining heterostasis is not essential for survival. The assumption is implicit that the maintenance of life is not necessarily the primary goal of all living systems.

Klopf proposes that the image of individual neurons being simply biological analogues of information-processing bureaucrats be replaced by an image of them being goal-seeking, adaptive units trying to establish a consensus of neural activity that primarily supports each individual neuron's needs and that allows intelligence to emerge as a by-product.

The inputs to each neuron are, in general, reinforcing and many of these inputs function as reinforcing feedback loops. There are approximately 10^{12} neurons exploring in parallel the consequences of activating 10^4 reinforcing feedback loops. Intelligent brain function can, therefore, be comprehended in terms of nested hierarchies of heterostatic goal-seeking adaptive loops, beginning at the level of the single neuron and extending upward to the level of the brain. To remind us of the social analogy, these multiple levels of heterostatic units would correspond to pleasure maximizing (actually, pleasure less pain maximizing) families, cities, and nations, for example. If we do equate pleasure with a neuron undergoing depolarization and pain with a neuron undergoing hyperpolarization, then pleasure and pain form the single bidirectional dimension to analyze mental phenomena. Their complex forms are identical with the spatial configurations of depolarizing and hyperpolarizing neurons.

2.7.1 Mathematical Model[6]

The neuron generates an action potential if

$$\sum_{i=1}^{n} w_i(t)f_i(t) \geq \theta(t_0),$$

where

$$
\begin{aligned}
n \quad &= \text{number of synaptic inputs to the neuron;} \\
w_i(t) \quad &= \text{synaptic transmittance associated with the ith input (exci-} \\
&\quad \text{tatory inputs have positive weights, inhibitory inputs have} \\
&\quad \text{negative weights);} \\
f_i(t) \quad &= \text{frequency measure of the input intensity at the ith synapse;} \\
\theta(t_0) \quad &= \text{neuronal threshold;} \\
t \quad &= \text{time; and} \\
t_0 \quad &= \text{time elapsed since the generation of the last action potential.}
\end{aligned}
$$

The heterostatic variable μ is maximized when heterostasis is achieved (i.e., the neuron experienced maximal polarization relative to environmental and adaptive mechanism induced constraints). Depolarization represents the positive aspect of polarization, hyperpolarization the negative. A neuron is in heterostasis for the time t to $t + \tau$ if the quantity $\mu_1^{t, t+\tau}$ is maximized:

[6]Adapted from Klopf, *The Hedonistic Neuron*, © 1982 Hemisphere Publishing Corporation. Reprinted with permission.

$$\mu_1^{t,t+\tau} = D_{t,t+\tau} - H_{t,t+\tau}$$

$$\Rightarrow \mu_1^{t,t+\tau} = \int_t^{t+\tau} (v_p(t) - v_r)\,dt - \int_t^{t+\tau} (v_n(t) - v_r)\,dt$$

$$\Rightarrow \mu_1^{t+\tau} = \int_t^{t+\tau} (v(t) - v_r)\,dt$$

where

$D_{t,t+\tau}$ = amount of depolarization experienced during t to $t + \tau$,
$H_{t,t+\tau}$ = amount of hyperpolarization experienced during t to $t + \tau$,
$v(t)$ = potential difference across the neuronal membrane,
v_r = neuronal resting potential,
$v_p(t)$ = $v(t)$ if $v(t) \geq v_r$, otherwise $v_p(t) = v_r$, and
$v_n(t)$ = $v(t)$ if $v(t) \leq v_r$, otherwise $v_n(t) = v_r$.

An alternative definition of the heterostatic variable that is more nearly attainable than the above one is as follows:

$$\mu_2 = E\left[\sum_{1=1}^{n} w_i(t)f_i(t)\right] \quad \text{and}$$

$$\Rightarrow \mu_2 = E[\alpha(t) - \beta(t)],$$

where

$$\alpha(t) = \sum_{i=1}^{m} w_i(t)f_i(t),$$

$$\beta(t) = -\sum_{i=m+1}^{n} w_i(t)f_i(t),$$

$[1 \leq i \leq m]$ = range of the numbered excitatory synapses,
$[(m + 1) \leq i \leq n]$ = range of the numbered inhibitory synapses,

and

$E[x]$ = expected value of x.

One possible adaptive mechanism in use here is described as follows. After the firing of a neuron, all excitatory and inhibitory synapses that were active during the process of determining whether the neuron should fire are eligible for channel transmittance changes. An eligible excitatory synapse has its channel transmittance increased if the generation of the action potential is followed by further depolarization for a limited time interval following the response, that is,

$$\left| \sum_{i=1}^{m} w_i(t) f_i(t) \right| > \left| \sum_{i=m+1}^{n} w_i(t) f_i(t) \right|.$$

Similarly the transmittance of an inhibitory synapse increases if the generation of the action potential is followed by hyperpolarization for a limited time interval following the response, that is,

$$\left| \sum_{i=1}^{m} w_i(t) f_i(t) \right| < \left| \sum_{i=m+1}^{n} w_i(t) f_i(t) \right|.$$

To put this adaptive process in the language of operant conditioning, let us call the input configuration s_t (which caused the neuron to fire) the neural conditioned stimulus (NCS) and let us call the stimuli s_{t+1} through s_{t+j}, received for a limited time interval after the NCS, the neural unconditioned stimulus (NUS). Klopf hypothesizes that the reinforcing effect of the NUS is maximal if it arrives approximately 400 ms after the NCS. (This is an extension of similar temporal relationships observed in Pavlovian conditioning.) Note that the only synapses whose transmittances are modified are those that played a role in transmitting the NCS. Synapses that transmitted the NUS do not have their transmittances modified even if they were also responsible for transmitting the NCS. The mechanism responsible for reinforcing this latter property is called *zerosetting*. Zerosetting plays a critical role in the model in that it prevents an input configuration from being reinforced merely by repeating itself. This suggests that neuronal reinforcement should result from the interaction of different subsets of synapses. Note also that under our implicit assumption that the stimuli arrive at discrete time intervals, there is nothing in the model to prevent a configuration serving as an NUS relative to a preceding configuration and as an NCS relative to a succeeding one.

A few remaining points regarding the heterostat are worth noting. The amount by which a particular synaptic transmittance changes depends on the delay between the NCS and the NUS and on the magnitude of the polarization throughout the effective reinforcement interval. Since the NUS could last as long as 4 seconds, it could consist of both depolarizing and hyperpolarizing input configurations. It is the relative amounts of each that then determine whether the NUS reinforces positively or negatively.

There are still some interesting questions regarding the heterostat that are as yet unanswered. For example, Klopf suggests that it is possible that instead of the entire neuron acting as a heterostat, limited areas of the soma and dendritic field act independently of one another from an adaptive standpoint. It is tempting to believe that synapses are reinforced only by other active synapses in the immediate area rather than by some located at a relatively greater distance, albeit associated with the same neuron. It is also likely that some neurons are nonadaptive and, if this is the case, these represent permanent constraints for the adaptive ones.

2.7.2 Comparison of the Heterostat with Alternative Neuronal Models

There are basically two types of connectionist neural models that have been employed in studying adaptive networks. The first of these is the *association model.* The principal tenet of the association model is that repetitive activation of a synapse, when this contributes to the firing of the recipient neuron, is the basis for increasing the effectiveness of the synapse. This is the oft-mentioned Hebbian rule. It is important to note that there is the assumption that adaptive changes are a function of co-occurring neuronal events. A classical conditioning orientation is implicit in such models.

The second kind of model is the *reinforcement model.* Here sequential rather than simultaneous events are of fundamental importance and an instrumental conditioning orientation is adopted. Adaptive changes are a function of reinforcement signals received after neuronal responses (in contrast with simultaneous events in association models).

Klopf points out that the Sutton-Barto thesis is a rejection of the Hebbian rule as inadequate. In general Klopf does not think that the association models are promising. Within the domain of reinforcement models, we have restricted reinforcement models (including the Widrow-Hoff model, which we investigate in Chapter 4) and generalized reinforcements models (including the heterostat). In the former, each neuron typically receives a few different signal types (different excitation and inhibition signals along with special reward and/or punishment inputs). The important thing to note here is that the reinforcement signals are of a special restricted nature, different in effect from the other inputs. Therefore there is a division between the source of the reinforcement signal, called the teacher, and the rest of the adaptive system. In the generalized reinforcement model, all (or many) input signals are potential reinforcers. There may be special teachers providing reinforcement, but environmental stimuli may do the teaching more directly.

Klopf provides a brief discussion of the primary points of departure of the heterostat from conventional adaptive network models. He argues that the conventional approach has been to devise network models on the basis of the overall system goals that the models were supposed to simulate (i.e., the tendency was to think top-down). In the heterostatic theory, a goal is assumed for the individual element and then the behavior of the total system is inferred from this elemental goal—a different perspective results. (Incidentally, the bottom-up approach also corresponds to the way in which living systems evolved.)

The heterostat also adopts a statistical adaptive process in which the chance occurrence of appropriate or inappropriate behavior is rewarded or punished. As the model that develops refines itself, the statistical aspect of the adaptive process becomes less critical. Other adaptive network research has assumed a deterministic adaptive process (e.g., Rosenblatt's perceptron convergence theorem uses an algorithmic adaptive procedure.) The difficulty with pure determinism is that of establishing what any given network element should be doing when the system behavior is inappropriate (not easy because the outputs of individual elements in a deep network are only highly indirectly related to the system's final output). We shall investigate the perceptron in Chapter 3.

Finally, it is interesting to note some of the implications of the heterostat for researchers in the AI field. They have conducted their research on grounds that are fundamentally different from researchers in the field of adaptive networks. While the latter have proceeded on the assumption that it is the individual neuronal level that holds the fundamental mechanisms underlying intelligence, the former do not regard that low a level as being one of any significance. This assumption displayed in Nilsson's (1974) survey of AI research (found in Klopf (1982)) is at odds with the heterostatic model that endows the individual neuron with the goal-seeking property.

> Knowledge about the structure and function of the neuron...is irrelevant to the kind of understanding of intelligence that we are seeking. So long as these components can perform some very simple logical operations, then it doesn't really matter whether they are neurons, relays, vacuum-tubes, transistors, or whatever.

Klopf suggests that there is a vast neuronal substrate, involving several levels of heterostatic reinforcing feedback loops, that has the potential to develop into a microscopic, nonlinguistic knowledge base. In bypassing the essential first step of microscopic-knowledge-base establishment and in proceeding directly to dealing with the linguistically oriented level, AI researchers could be making a mistake. Such an observation appears to be consistent not only with the evolutionary process (90 percent of the three billion years of life evolution has been spent in developing the neural substrate that we share with the reptile), but also with the fact that humans spend the early portions of their life developing microscopically detailed perceptions that are only very gradually shaped into abstract, higher-level views.

■ 2.8 Literature Overview

A good discussion on distributed representations is provided in Hinton (1986a). The idea of microfeatures and microinferences, mentioned in Section 2.2, is elaborated there along with a detailed discussion of the virtues of distributed representations. An interesting section deals with "coarse coding" and discusses the merits of dividing a space into several overlapping zones, assigning an identifier to each such zone, and then attempting to code features present in the space using these zones and their identifiers.

Kohonen (1972) provides a detailed discussion of correlation matrix memories, which were introduced in Section 2.4.3, and may be consulted for example applications of some of the theory presented in this section. Kohonen (1972) also provides an analysis similar to that described in this chapter, though slightly more complicated, for the ICMM case that results from the stochastic generation of connections without prior examination of the existing connections. Finally, the theory is applied to autoassociative correlation matrix memories (where a portion of the pattern constitutes the key) and to unsupervised learning in the ICMM case.

The material in Section 2.5 is drawn from Kohonen (1977). The paper emphasizes the importance of lateral inhibition in increasing the capacity and selectivity of a distributed network memory. A mathematical treatment of lateral inhibition is provided. The paper also reports a simulation in which one of 500 stored photographic images was recalled using a fraction of it as a key. There is, in general, more emphasis paid to the biological motivations for the model than is included in this chapter.

Kohonen (1979) and Kohonen (1983) may be consulted for far more complete treatments of associative memory.

Section 2.6 is a very summarized version of the Sutton-Barto theory. The reader can get a lot more by reading the source, Sutton (1981).

As mentioned in this book, the Sutton-Barto theory detects correlations between traces of stimuli and the output. A more detailed discussion of the consequences of such a model can be obtained from the paper.

Similarly, Section 2.7 provided only what was necessary to capture the essence of the Klopf thesis. The book, Klopf (1982), provides a much more comprehensive treatment of the theory and its ramifications.

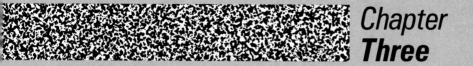

Chapter
Three

The Perceptron

■ *3.1 Introduction*

A *perceptron* is a net that undergoes training in the presence of supervision and is thus used as an associative memory. This chapter provides a survey of some of the important contributions in the literature regarding perceptrons and begins with a description of how Rosenblatt, the originator of perceptrons, envisioned its structure. Minsky (1969) discusses the inherently parallel nature of the perceptron's computation process. This is presented in the sections that follow along with discussions of the mathematics underlying the perceptron's decision processes, a presentation of the perceptron convergence theorem, and a comparison of the perceptron with other learning models.

■ *3.2 The Structure of a Perceptron*

Rosenblatt introduces the perceptron in the following manner.

> Perceptrons . . . are simplified networks, designed to permit the study of lawful relationships between the organization of a nerve net, the organization of its environment, and the "psychological" performances of which it is capable. Perceptrons might actually correspond to parts of more extended networks and biological systems; in this case, the results obtained will be directly applicable. More likely they represent extreme simplifications of the central nervous system, in which some properties are exaggerated and others suppressed. In this case, successive perturbations and refinements of the system may yield a closer approximation.
>
> Rosenblatt, *Principles of Neurodynamics*, 1962

The motivations for developing the perceptron model were as follows. Rosenblatt (1958) poses the following three questions as those most likely to provide the key to understanding the "mind."

1. How is information about the physical world sensed by the biological system?

2. What form is information stored, or remembered, in?

3. How does information contained in storage influence recognition and behavior?

The first question has been satisfactorily (for our purposes, at least) answered by physiologists; Rosenblatt's model seeks to address the latter two questions. The perceptron is a hypothetical nervous system that is designed to illustrate some of the fundamental properties of intelligent systems in general without paying attention to detailed mechanisms unique to particular organisms. The development of symbolic logic, digital computers, and switching theory has resulted in a spate of brain models that amount to specific algorithm executors in response to stimuli sequences. The premise of Rosenblatt's work is that imperfect neural networks, characterized by a plethora of random interconnections, cannot be appropriately represented by symbolic logic and Boolean algebra. The aim must be a mathematical analysis of the gross organizational structure; therefore, the perceptron is a probabilistic model, rather than one based on symbolic logic.

Earlier models that emphasised the study of deterministic approaches to perception and recall, as opposed to the study of actual brain mechanisms, failed in several respects. Rosenblatt mentions several, including absence of equipotentiality, lack of neuroeconomy, excessive specificity of connections and synchronization requirements, unrealistic specificity of stimuli sufficient for cell firing, postulation of variables or functional features with no known neurological correlates, and the like. Based on such shortcomings, Rosenblatt rejects earlier approaches in favor of his theory of statistical separability as illustrated in the perceptron.

Rosenblatt (1958) provides a description of a *photo-perceptron* (one that treats optical signals as stimuli), which is summarised here (see Fig. 3.1). Stimuli impinge on a retina of sensory S-points, each of which is assumed to respond on an all-or-nothing basis. These impulses are transmitted to a set of association A-units in a projection area A1. Each A-unit receives a number of connections from a collection of S-points; the latter are called that A-unit's origin points and these may be excitatory or inhibitory depending upon their effect on the A-unit. The A-unit

Figure 3.1 *Diagram of a photo-perceptron.*

From Rosenblatt, "The Perceptron: A Probabilistic Model for Information Storage and Organization in the Brain," Psychological Review, 65, No. 6, 386–408. © 1958.

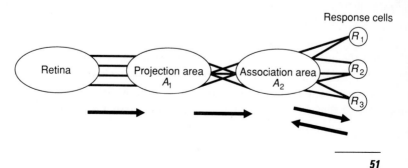

fires when the algebraic sum of excitatory and inhibitory impulse intensities is at least as great as that unit's threshold. The A-units in the projection area are randomly connected to more A-units in the association area, $A2$. The only manner in which projection A-units differ from association A-units is in their connection patterns. The last perceptron "layer" comprises a number of response cells, R, each of which has a large number of randomly located origin points in its source-set in $A2$. The R-units respond in much the same fashion as the A-units.

Feedback connections appear for the first time between the association $A2$ region and the response cells. Each response cell can have excitatory feedback connections to cells in its source-set or inhibitory feedback connections to the complement of its own source-set. Finally, note that the responses of such a system are mutually exclusive. Every response tends to inhibit not only all other responses but the source sets of all other responses also.

The impulses delivered by an A-unit will be characterized by a value, V. It is assumed that while the value of a particular A-unit is a fairly stable characteristic, it is increased during periods of activity. The logical characteristics of three different systems of value dynamics are displayed in Table 3.1. In the alpha system, an active cell gains an increment of value for every impulse. In the beta system, each source-set is allowed a certain constant gain-rate and the increments are apportioned among the source-set's cells in proportion to their activity. Finally, in the gamma system, in contrast to the alpha and beta systems, the total value of a source-set remains constant. The active cells gain in value at the expense of inactive cells.

Rosenblatt's detailed mathematical analysis of learning in the perceptron is thoroughly discussed in his paper. For the purposes of analysis, the system's response to a stimulus is assumed to occur in two phases. In the first, predominant phase, some proportion of A-units respond to the stimulus, while the R-units are inactive. In the second, postdominant phase, one of the responses becomes active and inhibits the activity of the other response cells. The initially dominant response cell is more or less random. However, repetitive presentations of the same stimulus cause the same response to have a progressively greater tendency to occur.

A deterioration in system performance occurs as the number of responses increases and the responses are all made mutually exclusive. One way of avoiding this deterioration is to find a limited number of discriminating binary features, each of which can be recognized as being present or absent in a particular stimulus and can therefore be represented by a mutually exclusive response cell pair.

Table 3.1 *Comparison of three value-dynamics systems.*

	α-system	β-system	γ-system
Total value gain of source-set per reinforcement	N_a	K	0
ΔV for A-units active for 1 unit	+1	K/N_a	+1
ΔV for inactive A-units outside of dominant set	0	K/N_a	0
ΔV for inactive A-units of dominant set	0	0	$-N_a/(N_A - N_a)$
Mean value of A-system	Increases with number of reinforcements	Increases with time	Constant
Difference between mean values of source-sets	Proportional to differences of reinforcement frequency $(n_{r1} - n_{r2})$	0	0

N_a = number of active units in source-set; N_A = total number of units in source-set; n_{rj} = number of stimuli associated to response rj; K = arbitrary constant.

Source: From Rosenblatt, "The Perceptron: A Probabilistic Model for Information Storage and Organization in the Brain," Psychological Review, 65, No. 6, 386–408. © 1958.

A perceptron with no capability for temporal pattern recognition is called a *momentary stimulus perceptron*. The same principles of statistical separability on which such a perceptron is based can be used to distinguish velocities and various sequences, provided the stimuli cause the activity in the A-units at a time t to depend on the activity at time $t - 1$. Rosenblatt also discusses other interesting modifications—for example, by suitable organization of origin points (as opposed to their random distribution), the A-units can be made to become particularly sensitive to contour location.

In recognizing the limitations of his model, Rosenblatt points out that the perceptron has no trouble learning responses to concrete stimuli. However, the model fails to recognize relationships between stimuli. Statistical separability cannot provide for higher order abstraction of relationships. While Hebbian physiology suggests the sort of organic substrate that might underlie behavior and attempts to show the plausibility of a bridge between biophysics and psychology, Rosenblatt's perceptron represents the first such completed bridge. The chief accomplishment of Rosenblatt's model might be summarized as follows.

> For a given mode of organization the fundamental phenomena of learning, perceptual discrimination and generalization can be predicted entirely from six basic physical parameters:
>
> x: the number of excitatory connections per A-unit
> y: the number of inhibitory connections per A-unit
> q: the expected threshold of an A-unit
> w: the proportion of R-units to which an A-unit is connected
> N_A: the number of A-units in the system
> N_R: the number of R-units in the system
>
> *From Rosenblatt, "The Perceptron: A Probabilistic Model for Information Storage and Organization in the Brain," Psychological Review, 65, No. 6, 386–408. © 1958.*

Note that each of these parameters is a clearly measurable physical variable, whose existence is not dependent on the phenomena that the perceptron is intended to model.

■ 3.3 The Parallel Nature of the Perceptron's Computation Process

The point stressed most often with regard to perceptrons by Minsky (1969) is that perceptrons make decisions—determine whether or not an event fits a certain pattern—by accumulating evidence from smaller experiments. Therefore, Minsky (1969) explores the simplest machines that are clearly parallel (because they have no loops or feedback paths), yet are capable of nontrivial computations. The simplest such parallel computation of a function, say, $\psi(X)$, is shown in Fig. 3.2. Essentially the functions

$$\phi_1(X), \phi_2(X), \ldots, \phi_n(X)$$

are computed independently of each other and combined by $\Omega(X)$ to produce the desired $\psi(X)$.

Now, if we take R to be the ordinary euclidean two-dimensional space, and X to be a geometric figure on R (X is to be thought of as simply a subset of the points of R), and if we let $\psi(X)$ be a function of figures X

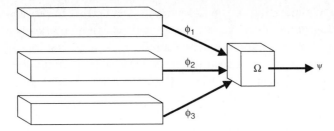

Figure 3.2 *Diagrammatic representation of parallel computation of a function.*

on R restricted to having two values, then we can define the notion of a predicate as follows. A predicate would simply be a variable statement whose truth or falsity depends on the choice of the figure X. Some examples of predicates would be

$$\psi_{convex}(X) = \begin{cases} 1 & \text{if } X \text{ is a convex figure} \\ 0 & \text{if } X \text{ is not a convex figure} \end{cases}$$

or

$$\psi_{connected}(X) = \begin{cases} 1 & \text{if } X \text{ is a connected figure} \\ 0 & \text{if } X \text{ is not a connected figure.} \end{cases}$$

We turn now to the concept of locality, which is important because locality of predicates allows their computation independently of one another. We define the convexity of a set X in the conventional manner: the set X fails to be convex if and only if there exist three points such that q is in the line segment joining p and r, and p is in X, q is not in X, r is in X. Then we can independently test all triplets of points and combine the results of these tests to determine whether the set X is convex or not. Now, we say that a predicate ψ is conjunctively local of order k if it can be computed by a set Φ of predicates ϕ such that each ϕ depends upon no more than k points of R:

$$\psi(X) = \begin{cases} 1 & \text{if } \phi(X) = 1 \text{ for every } \phi \text{ in } \Phi \\ 0 & \text{otherwise.} \end{cases}$$

The computation of the predicate ψ is supposed to proceed in two stages. Stage 1 involves the computation of many properties or features ϕ_α whose ease of computation is a result of their depending on only a small portion of R or is a result of some other elegant simplicity. Stage 2 involves a decision algorithm Ω that defines ψ by combining the results of Stage 1 computations. The division of the computation into these two stages would make sense only if Ω is distinctively homogeneous, or easy to compute. The perceptron scheme involves a definition for Stage 2 computations. Essentially, we are concerned with linear combinations of the predicates of Stage 1.

Let $\Phi = \{\phi_1, \phi_2, \ldots, \phi_n\}$ be a family of predicates. Then ψ is linear with respect to Φ if there exists a number θ and a set of numbers $\{\alpha_{\phi_1}, \alpha_{\phi_2}, \ldots, \alpha_{\phi_n}\}$ such that $\psi(X) = 1$ if and only if $\alpha_{\phi_1}\phi_1(X) + \ldots + \alpha_{\phi_n}\phi_n(X) > \theta$. Here θ is called the threshold and the α's are the coefficients or weights. Succinctly,

$$\psi(X) = 1 \qquad \text{if and only if } \sum_{\phi \in \Phi} \alpha_\phi \phi(X) > \theta.$$

Finally, Minsky (1969) defines a perceptron as a device capable of computing all predicates that are linear in some given set Φ of partial predicates. It is instructive to examine some of the categories that they find it useful to classify different perceptrons into.

1. *Diameter-limited perceptrons:* For each simple predicate ϕ in Φ, the set of points on which ϕ depends is restricted so as not to exceed a fixed diameter in the plane.

2. *Order-restricted perceptrons:* A perceptron has order less than or equal to n if no simple predicate depends on more than n points in R.

3. *Gamba perceptrons:* Each member of Φ may depend on all the points but must itself be computed by a perceptron of order 1 as defined in category 2.

4. *Random perceptrons:* The ϕ's are random Boolean functions and Φ is generated by a stochastic process according to an assigned distribution function.

5. *Bounded perceptrons:* Φ contains an infinite number of ϕ's, but all the α_ϕ lie in a finite set of numbers.

A few words of caution are appropriate. The idealised usage of the perceptron is summarised as follows. To make a perceptron recognize a particular pattern one merely has to set the coefficients α_ϕ to appropriate values. Such programs are representable as points $(\alpha_1, \ldots, \alpha_n)$ in n-dimensional space. Now it takes a small leap of imagination to devise a kind of automatic programming (which people have called learning). The perceptron is "programmed" by providing it with a series of input patterns and with a feedback device that generates an error signal to modify the coefficients whenever the perceptron responds inappropriately to any of its input patterns. The *perceptron convergence theorem,* covered in this chapter, defines conditions under which the perceptron is guaranteed to reach appropriate coefficients.

If Φ is the set of partial predicates of a perceptron and $L(\Phi)$ the set of all predicates linear in Φ, then $L(\Phi)$ is the perceptron's repertoire. Any physically realizable perceptron has a limited repertoire because for $L(\Phi)$ to be the set of all predicates, Φ would have to be very large. We now discuss some of the criticisms offered by Minsky (1969) of the manner in which perceptrons have been used.

Minsky (1969) argues that transforming geometrical classes of objects into n-dimensional vectors spawns a theory that is limited to counting the number of predicates in $L(\Phi)$. Intuitively simple predicates that belong to no practically realizable set $L(\Phi)$ are neglected. Conversely, some intuitively difficult predicates can be realized by low-order perceptrons (witness the example of ψ_{convex} mentioned earlier — this required only order 3 perceptrons).

Inadequate attention has been paid to the study of the information content and size of the coefficients. For example, sometimes the ratio of the largest to the smallest coefficient is hopelessly large or the information capacity needed to store the coefficients exceeds that needed to store the whole class of figures defined by the pattern.

On a related note, since practical perceptrons are finite-state devices, the perceptron convergence theorem is meaningless. Trivially, the perceptron could simply cycle through all possible states until the appropriate coefficients emerged. The question that is clearly relevant is the speed with which the perceptron learns relative to the speed of a random or an exhaustive procedure. Minsky (1969) has shown that, in some cases that are of geometric interest, the convergence time can increase even faster than exponentially with the size of the set R.

The point of this section is to emphasize that a perceptron whose predicates are properly designed for a discrimination known to be of suitably low order has a chance to improve its performance adaptively, whereas that is not the case when we give a high-order problem to a "universal" perceptron whose predicates are not at least somewhat task-specific.

Some flags of warning should also be raised against the temptation to get carried away with the notion of parallel programming. The critical tradeoff that is involved in choosing between parallel and serial methods of computation is whether the increased value of reducing the total elapsed time outweighs the cost of the additional computation involved. (To see how the total computation might be significantly greater than that in a serial process, consider that the parallel method requires that all the ϕ's be computed even though, in some cases, only a fraction of them are relevant to a decision.) All this points once again to the issue of locality. Minsky (1969) has shown that in some cases the vast number of partial functions with large supports (i.e., simple predicates depending on large subsets of R) dispels any hope that a modestly sized and randomly generated set of them would be dense enough to span the appropriate space of functions. The feasibility of consigning a problem to a parallel solution cannot be determined without determining the extent to which the problem can be split into local components.

■ *3.4 Basic Mathematics of Decision Surfaces*

The simplest case serves to illustrate the underlying principle adequately. A perceptron that decides whether an input belongs to one of two classes, A or B, can be a single node that computes a weighted sum of the inputs, subtracts a threshold, and passes the result through a hard-limiting nonlinearity such that an output of 1 indicates class A and an output of -1 indicates class B. Essentially, the perceptron forms two decision regions separated by a line (generalized to a hyperplane when we are dealing with more than two dimensions, i.e., when the number of classes is greater than two) whose equation depends on the connection weights and the threshold.

The relation of such functioning to associative memory should be clear. To continue with the above example, if instead of classifying an input as belonging to a particular class, we link it with a representative sample of the class, then whenever an input that even remotely resembles any of the classes is presented, the regenerated representative sample will be recalled.

The mathematical analysis of Duda (1973) underlying the theory of linear discriminant functions and decision surfaces forms the basis of

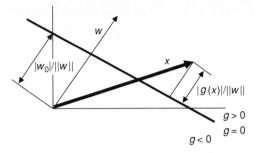

Figure 3.3 *The linear decision boundary g(x) = w'x + w₀ = 0.*

the perceptron's functioning (see Fig. 3.3) and is produced above to provide some insight into why the perceptron functions as it does.

3.4.1 The Linear Machine[1]

A discriminant function that is a linear combination of the components of x can be written as

$$g(x) = w^t x + w_0,$$

where

w = weight vector   and

w_0 = threshold weight .

A two-category decision classifier implements the following decision rule: decide ω_1 if $g(x) > 0$ and ω_2 if $g(x) < 0$. If x_1 and x_2 are both on the decision surface, then

$$w^t x_1 + w_0 = w^t x_2 + w_0,$$

$$\Rightarrow w^t(x_1 - x_2) = 0, \quad \text{and}$$

$\Rightarrow w$ is normal to any vector in the hyperplane.

[1]Text and figures from Duda and Hart, *Pattern Classification and Scene Analysis,* © 1973 John Wiley & Sons, Inc. Reprinted with permission.

In general, a linear discriminant function divides the feature space by a hyperplane decision surface whose orientation is determined by the normal vector w and whose location is determined by the threshold weight w_0.

The Linear Machine in the Multicategory Case. There are three different approaches to formulating decision surfaces in the multicategory case: (1) Reduce the problem to $c - 1$ two-class problems, where the ith problem's discriminant function decides whether or not a point is in ω_i. (2) Define $c(c - 1)/2$ linear discriminants, one for each pair of classes. Both of these approaches can lead to regions in which the classification is undefined. (3) Define c linear discriminant functions:

$$g_i(x) = w_i^t(x) + w_{i0} \qquad i = 1, \ldots c.$$

Assign x to ω_i if $g_i(x) > g_j(x)$ for all j not equal to i. This defines the *linear machine* and divides the feature space into c decision regions, leaving no areas in which the classification is undefined (see Fig. 3.4), with $g_i(x)$ being the largest discriminant if x is in region $\mathbb{R}_i$. Further, if $\mathbb{R}_i$ and $\mathbb{R}_j$ are contiguous, the boundary between them is a portion of the hyperplane H_{ij} defined by

$$g_i(x) = g_j(x)$$

$$\Rightarrow (w_i - w_j)^t x + (w_{io} - w_{jo}) = 0.$$

Clearly, $w_i - w_j$ is normal to H_{ij} and it is the differences of the weight vectors, rather than the weight vectors themselves, that are important.

The disadvantage of the linear machine is that the decision regions must be convex and singly connected. This limits the flexibility; in particular, the single-connectedness suggests that the linear machine is best used for problems having unimodal conditional densities $p(x/\omega_i)$.

The Two-Category Linearly Separable Case. Suppose n samples $\{y_i\}$ are to be classified into one of two categories. Suppose further that we have reason to believe that there exists a linear discriminant function $g(x) = a^t y$ for which the error probability is very low. A sample y_i is clas-

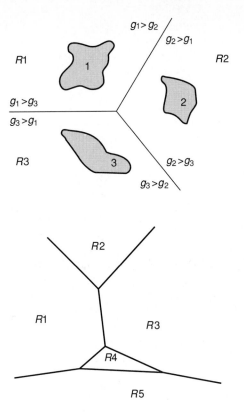

Figure 3.4 *Decision boundaries produced by a linear machine.*

A three-class problem is depicted in the *upper* figure. A five-class problem is depicted in the *lower* figure. In neither case are there any regions where the classification is undefined.

From Duda and Hart, Pattern Classification and Scene Analysis, *© 1973 John Wiley & Sons, Inc. Reprinted with permission.*

sified correctly if $a^t y_i > 0$, and y_i is labelled ω_1 or if $a^t y_i < 0$ and y_i is labelled ω_2. In the latter case, y_i is classified correctly if $a^t(-y_i) > 0$. Therefore we replace all ω_2 samples by their negatives and simply look for a weight vector a (the separating or solution vector) such that $a^t y_i > 0$ for all samples.

Each of the n inequalities specifies a half-plane and the solution region is therefore the intersection of n half-planes. Clearly, the solution vector (i.e., a) can lie anywhere within this region and is therefore not unique (Fig. 3.5). To prevent the possibility of the solution vector falling

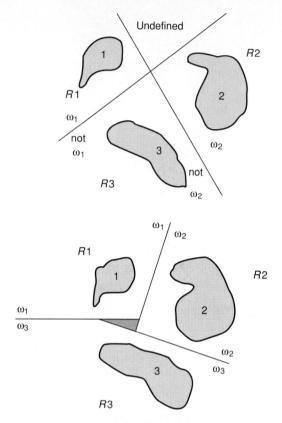

Figure 3.5 *Linear decision boundaries for a three-class problem.*

In the *upper* figure, the *i*th problem is solved by a linear discriminant function that separates points assigned to w_i from those not assigned to w_i. In the *lower* figure, we have a linear discriminant for every pair of classes. Both approaches leave regions where the classification is undefined.

From Duda and Hart, Pattern Classification and Scene Analysis, © *1973 John Wiley & Sons, Inc. Reprinted with permission.*

on the boundary of the region we might change the n inequalities to be of the form

$$a^t y_i \geq b > 0.$$

3.4.2 Gradient Descent Techniques[2]

Figure 3.6 illustrates the gradient-search technique for finding a solution region. We define a gradient descent vector $J(a)$ that is minimized when

---

[2]Text and figure from Duda and Hart, *Pattern Classification and Scene Analysis,* © 1973 John Wiley & Sons, Inc. Reprinted with permission.

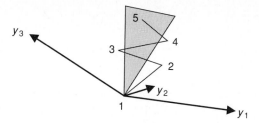

Figure 3.6 *Finding a solution region by a gradient search.*

The shaded region represents the solution space. Simply stated, the descent procedure is as follows: The next weight vector is obtained by adding some multiple of the sum of the misclassified samples to the present weight vector.

From Duda and Hart, Pattern Classification and Scene Analysis, *© 1973 John Wiley & Sons, Inc.*
Reprinted with permission.

an appropriate a is found. We start with some arbitrarily chosen weight vector a_1 and compute the gradient vector. The next value a_2 is obtained by moving some distance from a_1 in the direction of steepest descent (i.e., along the negative gradient). Therefore,

$$a_{k+1} = a_k - \rho_k \nabla J(a_k),$$

where

ρ_k = positive scale factor that sets the step size.

Small step size leads to very slow convergence, while large step size could cause overshoot and divergence. If the following approximation is valid,

$$J(a) \approx J(a_k) + \nabla J^t(a - a_k) + \frac{1}{2}(a - a_k)^t D(a - a_k),$$

where

D is the matrix $\dfrac{\partial^2 J}{\partial a_i \partial a_j}$ evaluated at $a = a_k$, then, combining the above two equations, we have

$$J(a_{k+1}) \approx J(a_k) - \rho_k \|\nabla J\|^2 + \frac{1}{2} \rho_k^2 \nabla J^t D \nabla J.$$

Therefore, to minimise the criterion function $J(a)$, choose

$$\rho_k = \frac{\|\nabla J\|^2}{\nabla J^t D \nabla J}.$$

■ 3.5 The Perceptron Convergence Theorem

Gradient descent techniques can be used to prove *Rosenblatt's perceptron convergence theorem* which states

> Given an elementary α-perceptron, a stimulus world W, and any classification $C(W)$ for which a solution exists; let all stimuli in W occur in any sequence, provided that each stimulus must re-occur in finite time; then beginning from an arbitrary initial state, an error correction procedure will always yield a solution to $C(W)$ in finite time
>
> Rosenblatt, *Principles of Neurodynamics*, 1962

Restated in the context of the present discussion, we have: if the inputs presented from two classes are separable (i.e., they fall on opposite sides of some hyperplane), then the perceptron convergence procedure converges and positions the decision hyperplane between those two classes. The original version of this procedure, described in Lippmann (1987), requires the connection weights and threshold values to be initialized to small random nonzero values. Connection weights are adapted only when an error occurs.

Minimize the perceptron criterion function,

$$J_p(a) = \sum_{y \in Y} (-a^t y)$$

where

$Y(a)$ is the set of samples misclassified by a.

Since $a^t y < 0$ if y is misclassified, the perceptron criterion function is always nonnegative. Since jth component of the gradient of J_p is $\partial J_p / \partial a_j$,

$$\nabla J_p = \sum_{y \in Y} (-y)$$

and

$$a_{k+1} = a_k + \rho_k \sum_{y \in Y_k} y,$$

where

Y_k is the set of samples misclassified by a_k.

The proof of the convergence of the perceptron criterion function lies in the following observation for single-sample correction (see Fig. 3.7). If a_k misclassifies y^k, then a_k is not on the positive side of the y^k hyperplane $a'y^k = 0$. The addition of y^k to a_k moves the weight vector toward this hyperplane (perhaps even crossing it). The new inner product $a_{k+1}^t y^k$ is larger than $a_k^t y^k$ by the amount $11y^k11^2$, and the correction is clearly moving the weight vector in a good direction.

We now provide a more mathematically complete treatment of the perceptron convergence theorem [Minsky (1969)]. Note that the ideas in this section have been presented earlier in this chapter.

Figure 3.7 *The basis of the perceptron convergence theorem.*

Since a_k misclassifies y^k, then a_k is not on the positive side of the y^k hyperplane $a'y^k = 0$. Adding y^k to a_k moves the weight vector toward this hyperplane.

From Duda and Hart, Pattern Classification and Scene Analysis, © *1973 John Wiley & Sons, Inc. Reprinted with permission.*

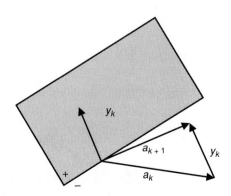

Let us assume that we wish to train a learning machine to respond YES to a stack of figures, called F^+, and NO to a stack called F^-. Assume further that the machine is a perceptron with a fixed Φ and adjustable coefficients. If a figure X, belonging to F^+, causes the sum

$$\sum \alpha_\phi \phi(X)$$

to be positive, or if a figure X, belonging to F^-, causes this sum to be negative, all is well. Any other response is incorrect and we are concerned with finding the simplest correction procedure for the perceptron. For convenience, let us think of the set of coefficients $\{\alpha_\phi\}$ as a vector in $|\Phi|$-dimensional space; similarly the values of the $\phi(X)$'s are the components of $\{\phi(X)\}$. Now we can use the notation $A \cdot \Phi$ instead of the usual summation, $\sum \alpha_\phi \phi(X)$. Now, consider the following program

START: Choose any value for A

TEST: Choose an X from $F^+ \cup F^-$
            If $X \in F^+$ and $A \cdot \Phi > 0$ go to TEST
            If $X \in F^+$ and $A \cdot \Phi \leq 0$ go to ADD
            If $X \in F^-$ and $A \cdot \Phi < 0$ go to TEST
            If $X \in F^-$ and $A \cdot \Phi \geq 0$ go to SUBTRACT

ADD: Replace A by $A + \Phi(X)$
            Go to TEST

SUBTRACT: Replace A by $A - \Phi(X)$
            Go to TEST

The perceptron convergence theorem simply states that regardless of the choice of START and TEST, the vector A will be changed only a finite number of times (i.e., A will eventually assume the value A^0 for which $A^0 \cdot \Phi(X)$ has the proper sign). To put this in terms of linear separability, the program listed above will separate F^+ and F^- if it is possible to do so. It is straightforward to note that the problem of finding a vector A to separate F^+ and F^- is the same as that of finding a vector A that satisfies

$$\Phi \in F \Rightarrow A \cdot \Phi > 0,$$

for a single F, defined as F^+ together with the negatives of F^-.

Then the convergence theorem may be restated as follows. Let F be a set of unit-length vectors. If there exists a unit vector A^* and a number $\delta > 0$ such that $A^* \cdot \Phi > \delta$ for all Φ in F, then the program

START: Set A to an arbitrary Φ of F

TEST: Choose an arbitrary Φ of F, and

        if A $\cdot$ Φ > 0 go to TEST

        otherwise go to ADD

ADD: Replace A by A + Φ

        Go to TEST

will go to ADD only a finite number of times.

A briefly sketched algebraic proof follows. Let

$$G(A) = \frac{A^* \cdot A}{|A|}.$$

Then, on successive passes through ADD, we have

$$
\begin{aligned}
A^* \cdot A_{t+1} &= A^* \cdot (A_t + \Phi) \\
&= A^* \cdot A_t + A^* \cdot \Phi \\
&\geq A^* \cdot A_t + \delta.
\end{aligned}
$$

We can say that the numerator of $G(A)$ increases linearly with n, since after n passes through ADD, we have

$$A^* \cdot A_n \geq n\delta.$$

Consider

$$
\begin{aligned}
|A_{t+1}|^2 &= A_{t+1} \cdot A_{t+1} \\
&= (A_t + \Phi) \cdot (A_t + \Phi) \\
&= |A_t|^2 + 2A_t \cdot \Phi + |\Phi|^2.
\end{aligned}
$$

For a pass through ADD to occur, $A_t \cdot \Phi$ must be negative. Therefore, the above expression is less than $|A_t|^2 + 1$. After n applications of ADD, $|A_n|^2 < n$.

Combining our results for the numerator and denominator of $G(A)$, we have

$$G(A_n) = \frac{A^* \cdot A_n}{|A_n|} > \frac{n\delta}{\sqrt{n}}.$$

Now, $G(A)$ is the cosine of the angle between A and A^*. Also $|A^*| = 1$. Therefore, $G(A)$ is less than or equal to 1. So, n must satisfy the relation

$$\sqrt{n}\,\delta \leq 1 \quad \text{or} \quad n \leq \frac{1}{\delta^2}.$$

Therefore, the process is finite.

There are two points to note regarding the above proof. First, we assume that each Φ repeats indefinitely often. Also, the final solution vector is not necessarily the same as A^*, the latter being an arbitrary solution vector. The set of solution vectors form a convex cone, A and A^*, are simply vectors within this cone.

Minsky (1969) describes several alternatives to the basic perceptron convergence theorem described above, all of which can be proved in a similar manner. One of the more interesting variations occurs when F is divided not just into the two classes F^+ and F^-, but into a multiplicity of classes. Let $F_1, F_2, \ldots$ be sets of figures and suppose that there are vectors A_i^* and $\delta > 0$ such that

$$\Phi \in F_i \Rightarrow \forall j \neq i, \qquad A_i^* \cdot \Phi > A_j^* \cdot \Phi + \delta.$$

Then the generalized theorem works in the following manner. Whenever one runs into a figure Φ in F_i for which $A_i \cdot \Phi < A_j \cdot \Phi$ for some j, A_i is increased and A_j decreased.

There are a couple of points worth noting about the perceptron convergence theorem in any of its forms. First, the statement "if two sets of figures are linearly separable then the theorem procedure can find a separating predicate" treats the perceptron as a mere homeostat. An enumerative procedure far simpler than the perceptron convergence theorem would suffice to find a separating hyperplane. Consider, for example, the following procedure,

START: Set $A_0 = 0$

TEST: Choose Φ from F
           If $A \cdot \Phi > 0$ go to TEST
           otherwise go to GENERATE

GENERATE: Replace A by T(A) where T is any transformation such that the series

T(0), T(T(0)), T(T(T(0))), . . . includes all possible integral vectors.

Go to TEST

Unlike the perceptron, this is a machine that does not profit from its experience at all—it is not a "learning machine."

The second important point is that convergence is guaranteed only when the sets (F^+ and F^- in the discussion above) are indeed linearly separable. This raises the question 'What happens to the vector A when this is not the case?' Clearly, there are practical reasons for studying the nonseparable case. One might, for example, wish to use the perceptron convergence procedure as a test for separability. Minsky (1969) shows, by proving the *perceptron cycling theorem*, that $|A|$ does indeed remain bounded. The cycling theorem essentially states that F-chains beginning with large vectors cannot grow much larger. Here an F-chain is a sequence of vectors $A_1, A_2, \ldots, A_n$ for which

$$A_{i+1} = A_i + \Phi_i,$$

$$\Phi_i \cdot A_i \leqq 0, \quad \text{and}$$

$$\Phi_i \text{ is an element of } F.$$

An F-chain is proper if

$$|A_i| \geq |A_1| \quad \forall\, i.$$

The cycling theorem can be stated as follows. For any $\varepsilon > 0$ there is a number $N = N(\varepsilon, F)$ such that if $A, \ldots, A'$ is a proper F-chain and $|A| > N$, then $|A'| < |A| + \varepsilon$. Note further that the lengths $|A|$ of the vectors are bounded. If the finite set of vectors in F are constrained to have integer coordinates, then the process is a finite-state one.

◼ 3.6 Scope of Decision Surface Methodology

Lippmann (1987) shows how a Gaussian classifier may be implemented using the perceptron structure. In fact, the decision regions formed by perceptrons are similar to those formed by Gaussian classifiers. Both these methods assume that inputs are uncorrelated and distributions for different classes differ only in mean values. The Gaussian classifier differs in making the strong assumption that the underlying distribution is

Gaussian. The perceptron training algorithm makes no assumptions concerning the shape of the underlying distribution; rather, it is concerned with the errors that occur when distributions overlap. Neither method is appropriate in the face of hyperplanar nonseparability.

There are clearly some serious limitations with the issue of hyperplanar separability. One problem is that decision boundaries may oscillate continuously when inputs are not separable and distributions overlap. In this case, a modification to the convergence procedure can form the least mean square solution. The resulting algorithm, called the *Widrow-Hoff method, delta rule,* or the *LMS (least mean square) solution,* is discussed in Chapter 4. Below is a summarised version of Lippmann's (1987) discussion of the choice of the number of layers and the number of nodes in a perceptron used to solve a particular problem (Fig. 3.8). It may be noted that while the discussion pertains to multilayer perceptrons with hard-limiting nonlinearities, a multilayer perceptron formed using sigmoidal nonlinearities (where we select the class corresponding to the output node with the largest output) can also be trained using a variant of the delta rule called the generalized delta rule of the backpropagation algorithm. The generalized delta rule is also discussed in Chapter 4.

A classic instance of classes not being separable by a hyperplane is the XOR problem. Distributions for the two classes for this problem are disjoint and cannot be separated by a single straight line. In the case of nonseparability of the inputs, we turn to the multilayered perceptron to solve this problem at least in some instances.

A *multilayered perceptron,* as its name suggests, has one or more layers separating the input and the output layers. Now, a single-layer perceptron forms half-plane decision region (i.e., the output of each node in the single layer specifies on which side of a particular hyperplane the input lies). In a two-layered perceptron, the nodes in the second layer take the intersection of the half-planes formed by the nodes in the first layer and can thus form any convex regions, including unbounded ones, in the input space. The number of the sides of the convex decision region is equal to the number of half-planes whose intersection formed the decision region. This provides an indication of how many nodes are needed in a two-layered perceptron. Specifically, the maximum number of sides of the convex decision region is bounded by the number of nodes in the input layer of the perceptron. To see how a three-layered perceptron can form arbitrarily complex decision regions, separate the desired decision region into small hypercubes. Now since hypercubes are convex, we can choose the first two layers of the perceptron such that the output of each

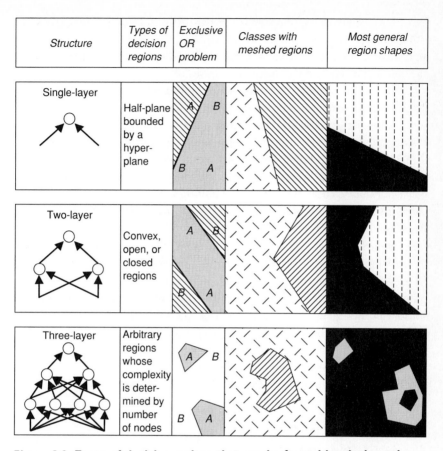

Structure	Types of decision regions	Exclusive OR problem	Classes with meshed regions	Most general region shapes
Single-layer	Half-plane bounded by a hyper-plane			
Two-layer	Convex, open, or closed regions			
Three-layer	Arbitrary regions whose complexity is deter-mined by number of nodes			

Figure 3.8 *Types of decision regions that can be formed by single- and multilayer perceptrons with one and two layers of hidden units and two inputs.*

Different shading is used to denote the decision regions for classes *A* and *B*. Smooth closed contours bound input distributions for classes *A* and *B*. Nodes in all nets use hard-limiting nonlinearities.

Reprinted with permission from R. Lippmann, "An Introduction to Computing with Neural Nets,"
IEEE ASSP Magazine, *April 1987. © 1987 IEEE.*

node in the second layer indicates whether the input lies in a particular hypercube. Finally, the hypercubes belonging to a particular decision region are brought together in the third layer. Each node in the third layer performs a logical OR of the inputs representing its decision region's hypercubes. Thus a node in the third layer will signal the presence of the input in the decision region that it represents if any of its hypercubes (represented by nodes in the second layer) indicate that the input is contained in them. Now, instead of hypercubes we could have used any other convex region. Clearly, the number of nodes in the second layer will have to be greater than one only if the decision regions are disconnected or meshed and cannot be contained in a convex region. In the worst case, the number of second-layer nodes must equal the number of disconnected decision regions required.

Note that increasing the number of layers in a perceptron only makes sense when nonlinearities are employed in the nodes. If the nodes of all layers implemented linear input/output characteristics, then characteristics of all the layers could be combined into a single linear characteristic. Finally, there is no point in having a perceptron with more than three layers as this is sufficient to generate arbitrarily complex decision regions.

In order to deal with the limitations mentioned above, it is critical to understand what is implied by *the capacity of a separating plane*. Consider the partitioning of a d-dimensional feature space by a hyperplane $w^t x + w_0 = 0$. Of the 2^n possible dichotomies of n d-dimensional sample points given in general position [i.e., no subset of $d + 1$ points falls in a $(d - 1)$-dimensional subspace], each labelled either ω_1 or ω_2, a certain fraction $f(n, d)$ are said to be linear dichotomies.

These are the labellings for which there exists a hyperplane separating ω_1 points from ω_2 points. This fraction[3] is given by

$$
f(n, d) = \begin{cases} 1 & n \le d + 1 \\ \dfrac{2}{2^n} \displaystyle\sum_{i=0}^{d} \binom{n - 1}{i} & n > d + 1. \end{cases}
$$

A graph of the above relation shows that a hyperplane is not overconstrained by the requirement of correctly classifying $d + 1$ or fewer points. It is not until n is a sizable fraction of $2(d + 1)$ that some difficulty arises. At $n = 2(d + 1)$, sometimes called the *capacity of the hyperplane*, half of the possible dichotomies are still linear. Thus, a linear discriminant is not effectively overdetermined until the number of samples is several times as large as the dimensionality.

A separating vector found for the design samples does not guarantee that the classifier will perform well on independent test data. This suggests that we use many samples to determine the hyperplane. However, the larger the data set, the less likely it is to be linearly separable. Thus we are faced with the need to compromise. The fixed increment

[3]From Duda and Hart, *Pattern Classification and Scene Analysis*, © 1973 John Wiley & Sons, Inc. Reprinted with permission.

(and some relaxation algorithms not elaborated here) algorithm that was mentioned above to motivate a proof for Rosenblatt's theorem is an example of an error-correction procedure because it modifies the weight only when an error is detected. There is, therefore, an implicit assumption that there does exist an error-free solution. It is worthwhile to reiterate that it makes sense to use such procedures only when the probability that there exists such a solution is high.

Two-layered associative networks (i.e., those possessing only an input and output layer with no intermediate hidden units), map similar input patterns to similar output patterns. Pattern similarity in a parallel distributed processing (PDP) system is determined by overlap, which in turn is determined by whatever produces the pattern (i.e., a source outside the learning system). The problem that Rumelhart (1986c) addresses is the failure of a network without internal representations (i.e., one without hidden units) to perform the mappings required when the representation provided by the outside world is such that the similarity structure of the input and output patterns are very different (e.g., in the XOR problem). The idea behind the hidden intermediate units is that there is always a recoding (i.e., an internal representation) of the input patterns in these units in which the similarity of the recoded patterns thus formed can support any required mapping from the input to the output units.

Recent work done by Baum (1988) on the capacity of perceptrons for computing dichotomies and on the ability of multilayer perceptrons to handle general input-output mappings is interesting, particularly from the theoretical point of view. These brief paragraphs are designed to convey a sense of the kinds of results that have been proved. Baum assumes the existence of a set S of N vectors in d dimensions and a function F into the e-dimensional hypercube, $F:S \rightarrow \{1, -1\}^e$. When $e = 1$ and the function F is simply assigning a value of $+1$ or -1 to the set S, we call F a dichotomy. Then it can be shown that the smallest multilayer perceptron capable of realising an arbitrary dichotomy on an arbitrary set of N points in general position in R^d is in fact a perceptron with only one hidden layer having $[(N - 1)/d + 1]$ internal units. N vectors in d-dimensional space are in general position if no subset of d or fewer vectors are linearly dependent. The only way to get a smaller multilayer perceptron is to adopt a stronger restriction on the set of N vectors. Naturally, this amounts to making the result less general.

Counting arguments can be used to derive lower bounds on the size of multilayer networks. A net with a hidden layer and synapses that could assume real values could perform better by a factor of $O(\log_2 (N))$ than a similar net with synapses that could only assume values along a "gray scale" (i.e., only a finite set of values). Counting arguments are also used to show that unless a multilayer perceptron has at least

$$O\left(\sqrt{\frac{N}{\log_2 N}}\right)$$

units, it cannot compute an arbitrary function, no matter how many layers it has. While these are questions of considerable theoretical interest, it is beyond the scope of this book to provide an analysis of the results. The Literature Overview section at the end of the chapter suggests further references for readers whose curiosity has been aroused.

While the perceptron convergence procedure (which we analysed above), or Widrow-Hoff's variation called the delta rule (presented in Chapter 4 in normal and generalized forms), provides a very simple guaranteed learning rule for all problems solvable without hidden units, it is important to note that no such rule exists for learning in networks with hidden units. As ennumerated by Rumelhart (1986c), there are three important responses to this lack:

1. *Competitive learning* employs simple, unsupervised learning rules, so that useful hidden units develop. No external force ensures that the units thus formed are appropriate.

2. *Interactive activation model* assumes an internal representation that, on some a priori grounds, seems reasonable.

3. *Boltzmann machines* develop a learning procedure capable of learning an internal representation.

A variation to the delta rule, the generalized delta rule, is described in Chapter 4. In the course of the next few chapters, in addition to examining the models mentioned above, we will also discuss the adaptive resonance paradigm, a variant of competitive learning.

■ 3.7 Comparison of the Perceptron with Other Learning Models

For the purpose of comparing the perceptron and its related convergence procedures with other learning machine models and their related procedures, Minsky (1969) proposes the diagram shown in Fig. 3.9.

Essentially, in the "finding" phase of its operation, the machine must decide which of a variety of n-dimensional query vectors belong to

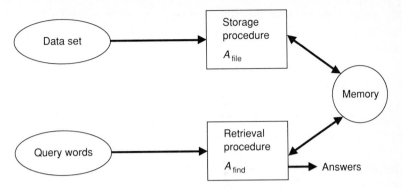

Figure 3.9 *Basic diagrammatic representation for information retrieval and inductive inference.*

the data set of n-dimensional vectors that were shown to the machine in its earlier "filing" phase. The algorithm that modifies the information in the machine's memory is called A_{file}, while A_{find} is the algorithm that decides the fate of the query vectors.

Minsky (1969) begins by comparing the perceptron to the machine called COMPLETE STORAGE. As its name implies, the machine merely stores all the elements of its data set in its memory in the order of arrival. Correspondingly, A_{find} simply performs exhaustive search on the contents of the memory. A simple comparison along several lines is instructive. First, COMPLETE STORAGE works on any data set, while the perceptron works only when the data set is linearly separable. Second, COMPLETE STORAGE needs a memory the size of the data set. The perceptron could have a summarizing effect when the storage required for its coefficients $\{\alpha_i\}$ is less than that required to store the input vectors, but this is not generally the case. Third, COMPLETE STORAGE's exhaustive search A_{find} is clearly slower than the perceptron's retrieval process. It is important to note, however, that if the former's A_{file} were modified to sort incoming vectors as they were stored into memory, then A_{find} could operate in $\log_2(|\text{data set}|)$ time. Finally, COMPLETE STORAGE could not operate if only a sample of the data set is shown to it, but perceptron might make a reasonable guess. Once again, a simple modification to the former makes it far more effective. Assuming continuity of the data set, we could have COMPLETE STORAGE's A_{find} simply return that point in its memory that is closest to the query vector. Under these circumstances, however, any speed up techniques (such as hash-coding) that would be possible if the entire data-set were in memory are no longer possible.

The salient points of this comparison are as follows. Both machines act incrementally, changing their internal representation of the data set as new data is presented, the change being a function not only of the most recently presented data element but also of the existing internal representation. Both machines operate in real time (i.e., without auxiliary memory) and neither machine assumes that the data will be presented to it in any particular order. Note, however, that the perceptron's A_{file} is based on feedback while COMPLETE STORAGE's A_{file} is very much a passive procedure. The cost of obtaining the feedback is that the former needs multiple presentations of the data set.

When the data set is divided into a number of classes $F_1, \ldots, F_k$ (as opposed to just two classes as assumed above — i.e., data is either in the set or out of it), the perceptron's A_{file} is presented with data-set members and also with the class to which that data belongs. Then A_{find} finds k vectors $A_1, \ldots, A_k$ and assigns the vector Φ to F_j if

$$\Phi \cdot A_j > \Phi \cdot A_i \qquad \forall\, i \neq j.$$

We can think of each F_j as a cluster of points in Φ-space and with each such cluster we can associate a point B_j that is the mean of all the vectors that we have observed in F_j. Then Φ is in that F_j for which the Euclidean distance $|\Phi - B_j|$ is the smallest. The set of points closer to a point B_i than to another point B_j is bounded by a hyperplane and hence is defined by a linear inequality. Therefore the two methods of assigning a class F_i to a vector Φ (i.e., the maximal inner product method and the nearness scheme) are essentially the same. By extension, the points closest to one of a number of B_j's forms a convex polygon that defines the set F_j.

Minsky (1969) suggests a variety of ways to divide up space into a number of classes. For each method, the same decision algorithm is used for A_{find}. Each class F_j has associated with it one or more A_i's; we say that A_i is associated with $F_{j(i)}$. For each vector Φ, choose that $F_{j(i)}$ for which $A_i \cdot \Phi$ is largest. For each model, A_{file} constructs the A_i's on the basis of prior information regarding the classes F_i or on the basis of prior experience. The first of these methods of space division is the perceptron procedure. Here, there is one vector A_j for each class F_j. The A_{file} procedure has already been discussed above.

In the Bayes linear statistical procedure, we again have one A_j for each class F_j. The A_{file}, which we discuss below, is quite different from that of the perceptron. The A_j's are chosen as follows. If, for each F_j and ϕ_i, we define

$$w_{ij} = \log\left(\frac{p_{ij}}{1 - p_{ij}}\right),$$

where

$$p_{ij} = \text{probability that } \phi_i = 1 \text{ given that } \Phi \in F_j,$$

then choose $A_j = (\theta_j, w_{1j}, w_{2j}, \ldots)$.

We digress a little from our earlier somewhat restrictive assumption that each Φ is associated with a unique F_j in order to elaborate on the bayesian method of space division. Generalizing, let us say that it is possible for a Φ to be associated with more than one F_j. Therefore, given an event Φ, we want to find that class F that is most likely to have produced that event. Now, if F_j is responsible for producing F, then we say that the joint event

$$F_j \wedge \Phi$$

has occurred, and by the laws of conditional probability,

$$P(F_j \wedge \Phi) = P(F_j) \cdot P\frac{\Phi}{F_j}.$$

Clearly, we have to choose that F_j for which the joint event is maximized. Further, we make an assumption about independence. Specifically, given that a Φ is in a certain class, no one or more of the partial predicates, ϕ, reveals any further information about the remaining ϕ values (i.e., the $\phi_i(X)$ are said to be statistically independent over each F-class). Therefore, we can elaborate on the above conditional probability as follows. For any $\Phi(X) = (\phi_1(X), \ldots, \phi_m(X))$, we say

$$P\frac{\Phi}{F_j} = P\frac{\Phi_1}{F_j}x \ldots xP\frac{\Phi_m}{F_j}.$$

Under this assumption of independence, define

$$p_j = P(F_j),$$

$$p_{ij} = P\left(\phi_i = \frac{1}{F_j}\right), \quad \text{and}$$

$$q_{ij} = 1 - p_{ij} = P\phi_i = \frac{0}{F_j}.$$

Then we want to maximize

$$p_j \cdot \prod_{\phi_i=1} p_{ij} \cdot \prod_{\phi_i=0} q_{ij} = p_j \cdot \prod_i p_{ij}^{\phi_i} \cdot q_{ij}^{(1-\phi_i)}$$

$$= p_j \cdot \prod_i \left(\frac{p_{ij}}{q_{ij}}\right)^{\phi_i} \cdot \prod_i q_{ij}.$$

This is the same as maximizing

$$\sum_i \phi_i \cdot \log\left(\frac{p_{ij}}{q_{ij}}\right) + \left(\log p_j + \sum_i \log q_{ij}\right),$$

and this can be written as

$$\sum w_{ij}\phi_i + \theta_j,$$

where

$$w_{ij} = \log\left(\frac{p_{ij}}{q_{ij}}\right)$$

and

$$\theta_j = \log p_j + \sum_i \log q_{ij}$$

and is independent of the presented Φ. Notice that this is clearly a linear threshold predicate. Therefore, the assumption of independence among the ϕ_i's leads to the linear decision policy.

It is instructive to compare the perceptron and Bayes procedures for space division. The Bayes procedure has a major advantage over the perceptron procedure in that it gives reasonable results for nonlinearly separable classes. Further, Minsky (1969) tells us that it gives the lowest possible error rate when A_{file} depends only on conditional probabilities (when the ϕ's are statistically independent as explained above). Minsky (1969) also provides some very basic geometrical sketches that illustrate the performance of these two schemes (Fig. 3.10). The Bayes line lies perpendicular to the line between the mean points of the two F classes. In the first case, the perceptron procedure eventually produces an appropriate hyperplane (no error) while in the second, it can do nothing since the classes are not linearly separable. Bayes, on the other hand, has a slight error in both cases.

Minsky (1969) also makes an interesting observation regarding an underlying assumption that must be made before any of the above discussion regarding linear separability and learning is to assume any relevance. We have inherently assumed that the F classes can be fit into some sort of collection of "clouds," for want of a better word, with some overlap (Fig. 3.11). Then there is an immediate difference between perceptron and Bayes that can be pointed out. The former is more concerned with the boundaries of these clouds, whereas Bayes weights all ϕ's equally.

Figure 3.10 *Comparison of perceptron and Bayes procedures for space division.*

From Minsky, Perceptrons: An Introduction to Computational Geometry, *Cambridge, Mass.:* The MIT Press. © 1969. Reprinted with permission.

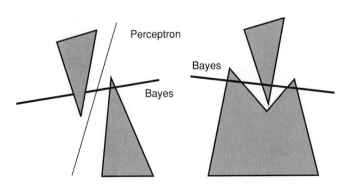

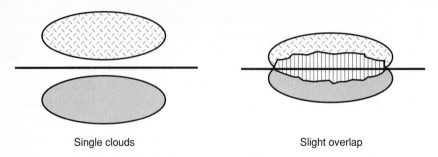

Single clouds   Slight overlap

Figure 3.11 *Assumed fit of F classes into "clouds."*

From Minsky, Perceptrons: An Introduction to Computational Geometry, *Cambridge, Mass.: The MIT Press.*
© *1969. Reprinted with permission.*

There are two other space division methods that Minsky (1969) discusses — *best plane* and *nearest neighbor.* The best plane scheme owes its conception to the fact that often, when the F_j's are not linearly separable, there will exist a set of A_j vectors that will perform better than those formed by either perceptron or Bayes. By definition, therefore, best plane is at least as good as perceptron or Bayes. Thinking in terms of clouds again, in cases that do not easily lend themselves to such classification, we can expect to see best plane outperforming both perceptron and Bayes because it is not subject to the bad influence of symmetry. Note, however, that best plane is subject to bad computation problems.

Nearest neighbor assumes no limit on the number of A-vectors. Very simply, A_{file} stores every single ϕ and its associated F-class. Then A_{find}, for any query vector, simply locates that stored Φ that is closest to the query vector and assigns its F-class to the query vector. Clearly, in the limiting case, this scheme works as well as any other. The most obvious disadvantage is the large memory requirement. Minsky (1969) points out that in some cases this scheme needs the sample size to be nearly the whole space before it can perform well. They show that nearest neighbor is worse than best plane, but not arbitrarily worse, and that this holds until enough points have been sampled that it is possible to say that the newly sampled point has been sampled before (i.e., the whole space is almost covered.)

Given a data set of information, Minsky (1969) seeks to investigate the space-time characteristics of various A_{file}-A_{find} combinations. Assume that we are given $2a$ binary words selected at random from a universe of $2b$ binary words (i.e., each of the words in our known data set is

b bits long). We want a machine that, when given a random b-digit word w, will tell us whether w is in the data set.

The machine has M bits of memory. When presented with the data set, A_{file} is expected to fill these M bits appropriately. Subsequently, neither the data set nor A_{file} are to be used again. A_{find} must answer the question posed above solely on the basis of the contents of the M-bit memory. Clearly, given M, we want to find an A_{file}-A_{find} pair such that the number of memory references made in answering the question is minimized. Minsky (1969) investigates several alternative approaches.

1. *Enormous Memory:*
   $M \geq 2^b$.
   A_{file}: set m_w to 1 if w is in the data set and A_{find}: w is in the data set if $m_w = 1$. Only one reference is required to answer the question.

2. *Inadequate Memory:*
   $M < (b - a)2^a$.
   Problem has no solution.

3. *Binary Logarithmic Sort:*
   $M = b \cdot 2^a$,
   that is, enough room to store the ordered data set. A_{file}: store the words of the data set in ascending numerical order and A_{find}: binary search to locate w. Requires a maximum of $\log_2 2^a = a$ inspections of b-bit words (i.e., $a \cdot b$ references).

4. *Exhaustive Search:*
   $M = (b - a) \cdot 2^a$,
   that is, enough memory to represent the unordered data set. A_{file}: Compute the successive differences of the words after putting them in numerical order. Use Huffman Coding to store this sequence, which should require about $(b - a) \cdot 2^a$ bits. A_{find}: Add successive differences in memory until the sum equals or exceeds w. w is in the data set only if equality occurs. This requires that we reference half the memory on average.

5. *Hash Coding:*
   $M = 2 \cdot b \ 2^a$,
   that is, twice the memory required to store the entire ordered data set.

Minsky (1969) shows that this simple doubling in memory (alternative 5) drastically reduces the number of memory references required if the technique of hash-coding is used to represent the data. There are several possible hashing schemes; the result of using the one proposed by Minsky (1969) is that one makes less than $2 \cdot b$ memory references on the average. While it is certainly true that particular hash-coding techniques might be especially unsuitable for specific data sets, the average behavior of any scheme on all possible data sets is certainly worth considering.

Now, it is very interesting to modify the questions a little bit and ask our machine to exhibit the word closest to w (query word) in the data set. Here, closest may be interpreted as having the smallest Hamming distance,

$$ d(w, \hat{w}) = \sum_{i=1}^{b} |x_i - \hat{x}_i|. $$

1. $M = 2^b \cdot b$.

   A_{file}: assigns for every possible word w a block of b bits that contains the appropriate bits of the correct $\hat{w}$. A_{find}: looks in the w block and writes out $\hat{w}$. This method uses b references.

2. $M < (b - a) \cdot 2^a$.

   Problem has no solution.

3. $M = b \cdot 2^a$.

   No known result.

4. $M = (b - a) \cdot 2^a$.

   This requires the same number of references as in the answer to our first question.

5. $(b - a) \cdot 2^a < M < b \cdot 2^b$.

   No useful known result.

Clearly, the results are rather disappointing for the second question (best match) as compared with those for the first question (exact match). For exact match, relatively small amounts of redundancy resulted in close to optimal serial computation. However, Minsky (1969) conjectures that even for the best A_{file}-A_{find} pairs in best match, there is little value obtained by allowing large memory redundancy.

■ 3.8 Literature Overview

There are a number of excellent literary references that supplement the material in this chapter. For starters, Lippmann (1987) provides a concise introduction to the notion of the perceptron. His paper, dealing with single-layered and multilayered perceptrons, is an excellent starting point. This paper has been used as a source for some of the discussion in Section 3.6.

Duda and Hart [Duda (1973)] have provided an excellent comprehensive text on pattern recognition. Section 3.4 merely scratches the surface of the techniques that are covered in their book. The latter covers techniques far beyond the scope of this book, but is nevertheless an excellent reference for anyone whose curiosity in pattern recognition is aroused. A lot of material can be found in their text to supplement Section 3.6 for example.

One of the main references for this chapter is clearly the classic work by Minsky and Papert [Minsky (1969)]. This has been cited extensively in this chapter and the reader is encouraged to consult the original text for supplementary material.

Baum (1988) is concerned more with the size of nets capable of realizing arbitrary or random functions than with the question of how a net might learn a structured function. Most of the paper deals with work on vectors topologically restricted to be in general position, but it shows that smaller nets can be used to realize arbitrary maps if the topological restrictions are relaxed somewhat. Baum (1989) addresses the issue of generalization versus size in networks. The principal result is: If the number of randomly chosen training examples from an arbitrary probability distribution is at least

$$O\left(\frac{W}{\varepsilon} \log \frac{N}{\varepsilon}\right), \qquad 0 < \varepsilon \leq \frac{1}{8},$$

then at least a fraction $(1 - \varepsilon/2)$ of future test examples from the same probability distribution will be correctly classified by a feedforward network of linear threshold functions with N nodes and W weights.

Another paper of theoretical interest that supplements the discussion in Section 3.6 is that by Cybenko (1989). This paper shows that arbitrary decision regions can be arbitrarily well approximated by continuous feedforward neural networks with one single hidden layer and any continuous sigmoidal nonlinearity.

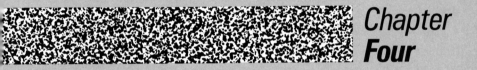

Chapter
Four

The Delta Rule and Learning by Back-Propagation

■ 4.1 Introduction

The *delta rule,* also called the Widrow-Hoff method or the LMS (least mean square) method, was mentioned in the discussion in Chapter 3 on the scope of decision surface methodology. In this chapter we describe the principles underlying the delta rule, noting especially that it is a gradient descent technique. A section is devoted to demonstrating how the delta rule can be extended from the case wherein there is a fixed target output pattern for each input pattern to the case wherein sets of input patterns are associated with sets of output patterns. The latter part of this chapter discusses the *generalized delta rule,* an extension to the delta rule, wherein learning proceeds by back-propagation of error signals. We have also provided a brief mention of applications of this learning paradigm and a discussion of the intractability of the network learning problem at the end of the chapter.

■ 4.2 The Delta Rule (Widrow-Hoff Rule)

The delta rule was first encountered in Section 1.2 of this book. From the form of the reinforcement signal mentioned there, it appears as though the rule functions by making corrections for errors, the corrections being determined by the teacher input $z(t)$. In fact, the rule is typically applied to the case in which pairs of patterns, consisting of an input pattern and a target output pattern, are to be associated. Imagine a situation in which the set of input/output pairs are repeatedly presented. Then the change in weight w_{ji} following pattern p is given by the product of the ith input element and the jth target element,

$$\Delta_p w_{ji} = t_{pj} i_{pi},$$

where

t_{pj} = desired or target output for jth element of pattern p and
i_{pi} = activation value of the ith element of the input for pattern p.

In vector notation,

$$\Delta_p = t_p i_p^T.$$

(If we assumed that this product rule is the sole criterion in determining the output unit's activation, then the rule is exactly the Hebbian rule.)

We have shown in a similar analysis that if the input vectors are orthonormal, then after the presentation of a series of P patterns, the weight matrix will be given by

$$W = \sum_{p=1}^{P} t_p i_p^T,$$

and subsequent presentation of any of the input patterns will result in the retrieval of the unique output.

4.2.1 Change of Basis[1]

What is, however, most fascinating about the delta rule is that it is not so much the contents of the specific patterns that matter as it is the pattern of correlations among the patterns. Stone (1986) substantiates this claim by changing the basis of representation from the unit basis to the pattern basis (Fig. 4.1). In an N-unit system, each pattern is represented by an N-dimensional vector whose elements represent the activations of each of the units (i.e., each unit is represented by one dimension). *Converting to the pattern basis involves transforming the coordinate system so that the*

Figure 4.1 *Conversion from unit-based coordinates into pattern-based coordinates.*

From Stone, "An Analysis of the Delta Rule and the Learning of Statistical Associations," in Rumelhart (ed.), Parallel Distributed Processing, Explorations in the Microstructure of Cognition, Vol. 1: Foundations, *Cambridge, Mass.: The MIT Press, 1986. Reprinted with permission.*

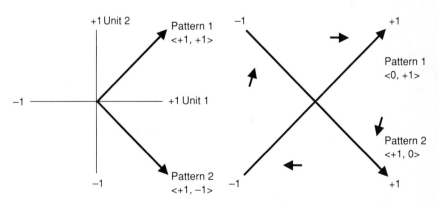

[1]Math in Section 4.2.1 from Stone, "An Analysis of the Delta Rule and the Learning of Statistical Associations," in Rumelhart (ed.), *Parallel Distributed Processing, Explorations in the Microstructure of Cognition, Vol. 1: Foundations,* Cambridge, Mass. The MIT Press, 1986. Reprinted with permission.

patterns line up with the axes. Now each pattern is represented by one dimension.

We need two transformation matrices: P_I that transforms the input patterns into a space based on the input patterns and P_T that transforms the output patterns into a space based on the output patterns.

For input vectors,

$$i_i^* = P_I i_i.$$

For target vectors,

$$t_i^* = P_T t_i.$$

For output vectors,

$$o_i^* = P_T o_i.$$

To derive the weight matrix under the new coordinate system, recall that in the old bases $Wi = o$. Therefore, we should now be able to write $W^* i^* = o^*$. Therefore,

$$W^* P_I i = P_T o,$$

$$\Rightarrow P_T^{-1} W^* P_I i = o = Wi, \quad \text{and}$$

$$\Rightarrow W^* = P_T W P_I^{-1}.$$

The rule in the old coordinate system that determined the updated weight matrix when a new (assumed orthonormal) input pattern was presented,

$$W(n) = W(n - 1) + \eta \delta(n) i^T(n),$$

where

$W(n)$ = state of the weight matrix after n presentations,
$i(n)$ = input presented on the nth presentation, and
$\delta(n)$ = $t(n) - W(n - 1)i(n)$, that is, the difference between the desired and actual output on trial n,

now becomes (when multiplied on the left by P_T and on the right by P_I^{-1})

$$P_T W P_I^{-1}(n) = P_T W P_I^{-1}(n-1) + P_T \eta \delta(n) i^T(n) P_I^{-1}$$

$$\Rightarrow W^*(n) = W^*(n-1) + \eta \delta^*(n) [P_I^{-1} i^*(n)]^T P_I^{-1},$$

where

$$\delta^*(n) = t^*(n) - W^*(n-1) i^*(n),$$

and finally,

$$W^*(n) = W^*(n-1) + \eta \delta^*(n) i^*(n)^T C,$$

where

$$C = (P_I^{-1})^T P_I^{-1}.$$

C holds the correlational information among the original input patterns.

The output vectors in the new basis have a very useful interpretation. *The jth component of an output vector represents the amount of the jth pattern found in the output.* This leads very naturally to the definition of error in such a system,

$$E_p = \sum_j (t_j^* - o_j^*).$$

4.2.2 Gradient Descent in the Ordinary Delta Rule[2]

The proposed learning procedure depends on the presentation of a set of pairs of input and output patterns. Learning (i.e., weight modification) occurs only when the output generated by the network in response to the input does not match the output provided in the pair. The rule used for weight changing following i/o pair p is

$$\Delta_p w_{ji} = \eta(t_{pj} - o_{pj}) i_{pi} = \eta \delta_{pj} i_{pi},$$

---

[2]Math in Section 4.2.2 from Stone, "An Analysis of the Delta Rule and the Learning of Statistical Associations," in Rumelhart (eds.), *Parallel Distributed Processing, Explorations in the Microstructure of Cognition, Vol. 1: Foundations,* Cambridge, Mass.: The MIT Press, 1986. Reprinted with permission.

where

t_{pj} = jth component of the output produced by the net,
o_{pj} = jth component of the actual output pattern, and
i_{pi} = ith component of the input pattern.

The delta rule minimizes the squares of the differences between the actual and the desired output values summed over the output units and all pairs of input/output vectors. A cursory outline of the proof is given in this summary. Let

$$E_p = \frac{1}{2} \sum_j (t_{pj} - o_{pj})^2$$

be a measure of the error on input/output pattern p and let $E = \Sigma E_p$ be the overall measure. The proof shows that the delta rule implements a gradient descent in E when the units are linear. This corresponds to performing steepest descent on a surface in weight space whose height at any point in weight space is equal to the error measure. It is shown that

$$-\frac{\partial E_p}{\partial w_{ji}} = \delta_{pj} i_{pi} \propto \Delta_p w_{ji}.$$

Combining this with the observation that

$$\frac{\partial E}{\partial w_{ji}} = \sum_p \frac{\partial E_p}{\partial w_{ji}}$$

Rumelhart (1986c) concludes that the net change in w_{ji} after one complete cycle of pattern presentations is proportional to this derivative, and hence that the delta rule implements a gradient descent in E and thus minimizes the error function.

4.2.3 Extension of the Delta Rule to Statistical Learning[3]

Instead of associating particular pairs of patterns, let us associate pairs of categories of patterns (i.e., the input/output pairs of patterns will be

---

[3]Math in Section 4.2.3 from Stone, "An Analysis of the Delta Rule and the Learning of Statistical Associations," in Rumelhart (ed.), *Parallel Distributed Processing, Explorations in the Microstructure of Cognition, Vol. 1: Foundations*, Cambridge, Mass.: The MIT Press, 1986. Reprinted with permission.

treated as random variables). Thus, when we pick the jth pair, input patterns i_j and target pattern t_j can take on random values. The ensuing analysis, provided by Stone (1986), holds regardless of the underlying distributions of these random variables. We also expect all the input/output pairs to be governed by some probability distribution. None of these distributions should change with time. If we start with the by now familiar form of the delta rule,

$$W(n) = W(n - 1) + \eta[t(n) - W(n - 1) \cdot i(n)] \cdot i^T(n),$$

and take expected values on both sides, we have

$$E[W(n)] = E[W(n - 1)](I - \eta E[i(n) \cdot i^T(n)]) + \eta E[t(n) \cdot i^T(n)].$$

Assuming that each selection of an input/output pair is independent of all previous selections, we can say that

$$E[W(n - 1) \cdot i(n)i^T(n)] = E[W(n - 1)] \cdot E[i(n) \cdot i^T(n)].$$

If $R_I = E[ii^T]$ and $R_{IO} = E[ti^T]$ represent, respectively, the statistical correlations among the input patterns and the statistical correlations between the input and target patterns, we can rewrite our previous result as

$$E[W(n)] = E[W(n - 1)](I - \eta R_I) + \eta R_{IO}.$$

Now, if we solve this recursive relation with the assumption that we started with an empty weight matrix (i.e., $W(0) = 0$), then we have

$$E[W(n)] = \eta R_{IO} \sum_{j=0}^{j=n} (I - \eta R_I)^j.$$

Recall that the pseudo-inverse of a matrix B, called B^+, is given by

$$B^+ = \eta B^T \sum_{j=1}^{\infty} (I - \eta BB^T)^j.$$

Since R_I has independent rows and columns, we can select a P with independent rows and columns such that $PP^T = R_I$. Note that P satisfies

$$(P^T)^{-1}P^T = I.$$

In the limit $E[W(n)]$ satisfies the following relation

$$\lim_{n \to \infty} E[W(n)] = E[W_\infty] = R_{IO}(P^T)^{-1}\left[\eta P^T \sum_{j=1}^{\infty} (I - \eta P P^T)^j\right],$$

substitute for the pseudo-inverse of P to get

$$E[W_\infty] = R_{IO}(P^T)^{-1}P^+ = R_{IO}(PP^T)^{-1} = R_{IO}R_I^{-1} = R_{IO}R_I^+.$$

Now, investigate what happens when the system is presented with an input i. Proceeding on our usual assumption of independence, we have

$$E[W_\infty i] = E[W_\infty]E[i],$$

$$\Rightarrow E[W_\infty i] = R_{IO}R_I^+ E[i] = E[ti^T(ii^T)^+]E[i],$$

$$\Rightarrow E[W_\infty i] = E[t(i^+i)^T(i^+i)], \quad \text{and}$$

$$\Rightarrow E[W_\infty i] = E[t],$$

which is the required result. Note above that we have used the relation $(AB)^+ = B^+A^+$, which is true when $A = i$, $B = i^+$, and i is a column vector. Further, $i^+i = 1$ since i has only one column.

This shows that the average response to inputs is equal to the average of the target patterns. This would imply that the expected response to a particular pattern will be the expected value of the target as long as the i and t patterns are distributed normally with zero means. It is not difficult to convert a set of input vectors into a set of zero mean patterns, nor is the requirement of normal distribution very restrictive when the patterns are of large dimensionality and are themselves the output of a linear system.

■ 4.3 The Generalized Delta Rule: Learning by Back-Propagation

For the case that we have discussed (i.e., using a linear activation function in a network with only an input and an output layer), the error surface is very conveniently shaped like a bowl. Consequently, gradient descent is sure to find the single minimum error set of weights. With hidden units, derivative-computation is not obvious and there is the danger of getting stuck at a local minimum on the complicated error surface. Rumelhart (1986c) shows that there does indeed exist a way of finding the "elusive" derivatives and that the problem of local minima is irrelevant in a wide variety of learning tasks. We shall have more to say about the necessity of relying on a methodology that will fail in the worst case in the section dealing with the intractability of the network learning problem.

For the purposes of studying simple learning by back-propagation, consider a layered feedforward network with a semilinear activation function. A layered feedforward network is specified by the following characteristics. The bottom and top layers are for input and output, respectively. Every unit receives inputs from layers lower than its own and must send output to layers higher than its own. Given an input vector, the output vector is computed by a forward pass that computes the activity levels of each layer in turn, using the already computed activity levels in the earlier layers. An example of a simple feedforward net is shown in Fig. 4.2.

A semilinear activation function is one in which the output of a unit is a nondecreasing and differentiable function of the net total output, $net_{pj} = \Sigma_i w_{ji} o_{pi}$. That is, for such a function

$$o_{pj} = f_j(net_{pj}),$$

where f is differentiable and nondecreasing. It is worth emphasising that it does not make sense to have hidden units with linear activation functions since any combination of linear functions can be combined into a linear function, thus eliminating any justification for having a separate layer.

Figure 4.2 *Simple feedforward net.*

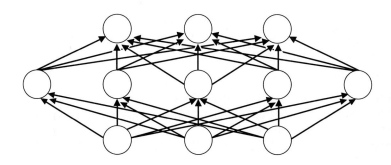

The proof of the generalized delta rule involves a more elaborate version of the reasoning outlined in the proof of the delta rule. The results that emerge from the proof are:[4]

→ The generalized rule has the same form as the standard version—that is, the weight on each line should be changed by an amount proportional to the product of an error signal δ, available to the unit receiving input along that line and the output of the unit sending activation along that line

$$\Delta_p w_{ji} = \eta \delta_{pj} o_{pi}.$$

→ There are two other equations that specify the error signal. For output units, the error signal is very similar to the standard delta rule and is given by

$$\delta_{pj} = (t_{pj} - o_{pj}) f_j'(\text{net}_{pj}),$$

where f_j is the semilinear activation function that maps the total input to the unit to an output value. The error signal for hidden units for which there is no specified target is determined recursively in terms of those of the units to which it directly connects and the weights of those connections, that is,

$$\delta_{pj} = f_j'(\text{net}_{pj}) \sum_k \delta_{pk} w_{kj}.$$

The generalized rule is applied in two phases. First, the output value o_{pj} is computed for each unit. This is then compared with the targets (i.e., the output provided as part of the i/o pair) and an error signal δ_{pj} results for each output unit. In the second phase (whose computational complexity is the same as that for the first phase) a backward pass allows the recursive computation for δ as indicated by the equations above.

---

[4] From Rumelhart, "Learning Internal Representations by Error Propagation," in Rumelhart (ed.), *Parallel Distributed Processing, Explorations in the Microstructure of Cognition, Vol. 1: Foundations,* Cambridge, Mass.: The MIT Press, 1986. Reprinted with permission.

Note that the linear threshold function, on which the perceptron is based, is discontinuous — its derivative does not exist and hence it cannot be used for the generalized delta rule. Instead we use the logistic activation function

$$o_{pj} = \frac{1}{1 - e^{-\left(\sum_i w_{ji} o_{pi} + \theta_j\right)}},$$

where

θ_j = bias similar in function to a threshold.

Not only is the derivative of this function easy to compute, it has an additional advantage. We can show that the derivative of o_{pj} with respect to total input, net_{pj}, reaches its maximum when $o_{pj} = 0.5$ and its minimum as o_{pj} approaches 0 or 1. [Note that $0 <= o_{pj} <= 1$] Since the weight change is proportional to the derivative, maximum change occurs for those units near their midrange, that is, for those units that are not yet committed to being either on or off. This feature contributes to the system stability.

There is a point to be made regarding some of the terminology that we have been employing. In a strict gradient descent, we would modify a particular weight w_{ji} only after we had determined the true direction of steepest descent. Now, this true direction is determined by the vector sum of directions of descent suggested by the presentation of individual patterns in the ensemble

$$\frac{\delta E}{\delta w_{ji}} = \sum_p \frac{\delta E_p}{\partial w_{ji}}.$$

Since the process described above changes the weight w_{ji} after each presentation of a pattern, rather than after the presentation of a complete cycle of patterns, the resultant descent in weight space is not necessarily the steepest. However, as long as the weight changes at any instant are not too large, the approximation to steepest descent is valid. This can be ensured by using a small learning rate, η. Shown in Fig. 4.3 is a simple diagram illustrating this point. Here, the pattern ensemble is composed of only two patterns, p_1 and p_2. The process described above causes descent to occur along the directions suggested by the individual patterns rather than along that of steepest descent.

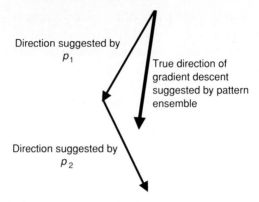

Figure 4.3 *Relationship between the directions of descent suggested by individual patterns and of that suggested by the pattern ensemble.*

The magnitude in weight changes is determined in part by the constant of learning, η. We would like this to be as high as possible without inviting oscillatory phenomena during descent along some "unfriendly" surfaces. One way to implement a reduction in such phenomena is to introduce a momentum term that gives some importance to past weight changes on the current weight change being considered:

$$\Delta w_{ji}(n + 1) = \eta(\delta_{pj}o_{pi}) + \alpha\Delta w_{ji}(n),$$

where

      n = presentation number,
      η = learning rate, and
      α = constant that determines the effect of past weight changes on the current direction of movement in weight space.

Remember that true gradient descent would require that the learning rate be infinitesimally small (i.e., the movement in weight space after every ensemble presentation be extremely small and in the direction of the gradient vector). Experiments have shown that a faster way to achieve the results brought about by a small learning rate is to use a large learning rate, η, in conjunction with a large momentum factor, α.

■ *4.4 Applications of Learning by Back-Propagation*

The back-propagation paradigm has been tested in numerous applications including bond rating, mortgage application evaluation, protein structure determination, backgammon playing, and handwritten digit recognition. To get a flavor of the general applicability of this paradigm, we have provided a very brief discussion of one of these applications below.

4.4.1 Bond Rating

Bond rating refers to the process by which a particular bond is assigned a label that categorizes the ability of the bond's issuer to repay the coupon and par value of that bond. Thus, for example, the Standard and Poor's organization might assign a rating varying from AAA (very high probability of payment) to BBB (possibility of default in times of economic adversity) for investment grade bonds. The problem here is that there is no hard and fast rule for determining these ratings. Rating agencies must consider a vast spectrum of factors before assigning a rating to an issuer. Some of these factors, such as sales, assets, liabilities, and the like, might be well defined. Others such as willingness to repay are quite nebulous. Thus a precise problem definition is not possible.

Dutta (1988) maintains that problems with nonconservative domains (the class of problem domains that lack a domain model) such as that seen in the bond-rating problem could be better solved by training a network using back-propagation than by trying to perform a statistical regression. The latter is inappropriate because it is unclear what factors the regression should be performed with, that is, it is not clear what factors the dependent variable (the default risk) really depends on. They describe details of experiments that they conducted with networks having no hidden layers and with networks with one hidden layer (with different numbers of nodes in the hidden layer). Bond ratings for 30 companies together with ten financial variables were used as data in the training of the neural network using back-propagation. The network was then used to predict the ratings of seventeen other issuers and consistently outperformed standard statistical regression techniques.

■ *4.5 Intractability of Network Learning*

Learning by back-propagation has been quite successful when applied to specific problems. Nevertheless, it is a problem whose worst case results in failure (this corresponds to getting trapped in a local minimum during gradient descent). This raises the very important question of whether there is an efficient general solution to learning in feedforward networks. Just such a question has been addressed by Judd (1987).

Let us digress for a moment and talk briefly about intractability. The first important distinction is between polynomial time and exponential time algorithms. An algorithm operates in polynomial time if its time complexity function is $O(p(n))$, where p is some polynomial function of the input size n. We cannot express a bound on the time complexity of an exponential time algorithm. The next important distinction is between the classes P and NP. A problem is in P if there exists a deterministic algorithm that solves it in polynomial time. In contrast, it is in NP if there exists a nondeterministic algorithm that solves it in polynomial time. This latter statement requires some clarification. As Garey (1979) explains, a nondeterministic algorithm is best viewed as one operating in two stages — a guessing stage and a checking stage. The first stage guesses a solution to the problem and the second checks, in a normal deterministic manner, to see whether the solution is appropriate. It is important to note that the checking stage operates in polynomial time. Clearly, any problem in P is also in NP. The outstanding problem of the day is whether this inclusion of P in NP is proper (i.e., does $P = NP$)? Though it has not been proven, the present thinking is that P does not include NP. Finally, NP-complete problems are the hardest problems in NP. If a particular problem is NP-complete, then every instance of every problem in NP can be converted to an instance of this particular problem and this conversion can be effected in polynomial time. This suggests that the solution of any NP-complete problem would result in the solution of all problems in NP.

With that brief discussion as background, let us return to neural nets. The problem being tested for NP-completeness is one of supervised learning in a nonrecurrent (hitherto referred to as feedforward) network. The aim is basically to get the network to memorize training data in the form of stimulus and response strings and subsequently to respond to any one of the stimulus strings by emitting its corresponding response string. Now, though this does not address the issue of generalizing the training data, this problem does prove to be NP-complete, which implies the intractability of the more general problem of generalizing from regularities inferred from the training patterns.

Though we shall not delve into the proof itself, it is instructive to consider the manner in which the problem is constructed. The functions performed by a particular network are the composite function of those performed by the individual nodes that comprise the network. Now, if a particular network is given the task of memorizing a set of stimulus-response pairs, the problem is to find a composite function (by finding the individual functions that the nodes should compute) that allows the task to be "loaded" onto the architecture. Clearly, *loading* is the process by which an appropriate function is specified for every node. As a measure of problem size, let the size be given by the number of nodes in the network plus the total number of bits in the stimulus-response pairs of strings. The implication of this problem being *NP*-complete is that the expression that determines the number of computation steps needed to effectively load a particular task onto a particular network is an exponential function of the problem size. Therefore, there is no single purpose general algorithm that will efficiently load an arbitrary task onto an arbitrary architecture in polynomial time.

This is not as discouraging as it sounds. Remember that most of the successes in the field have been derived from the consideration of very specific architectures and/or very specific tasks. So the fact that there is no single algorithm that does essentially everything that connectionism ever set out to accomplish is not really that surprising. Future research might show the existence of some sort of middle ground more general than dealing with specific instances of the loading problem and not as general as the complete loading problem. Also note that time complexity, on which the entire discussion of *NP*-completeness is based, is a worst-case measure, which means that it might well be the case that though an algorithm has very poor worst-case performance predictions, it might work very well for most problem instances (the simplex algorithm is a case in point).

■ *4.6 Literature Overview*

The mathematical results in Sections 4.2.1 and 4.2.3 are from Stone (1986). This reference provides an example showing conversion from unit-based to pattern-based coordinates, and a discussion showing the link between the delta rule and multiple linear regression.

The summarised derivations of gradient descent in Sections 4.2.2 and 4.3 are from a paper by Rumelhart (1986c). This paper provides several examples of the use of the learning-by-back-propagation algorithm, including a discussion of the parity and encoding problems. While the discussion in this book has confined itself to feedforward nets of the kind described in Section 4.3, it turns out that this learning algorithm applies to a more general class of recurrent nets — an introduction can be found in Rumelhart (1986c).

Judd's (1987) paper provides the intractability arguments presented in this chapter. For those familiar with the techniques used to prove that particular problems are *NP*-complete, the proof of the *NP*-completeness of the loading problem is done by reduction from SAT. The paper also presents and then refutes several arguments that might be presented to detract from the proof of *NP*-completeness of the problem.

For those intrigued by the notion of *NP*-completeness and the tantalizing question, does $P = NP$, Garey and Johnson provide an excellent discussion of intractability [Garey (1979)]. The first chapter of Garey (1979) provides an informal discussion of the significance of *NP*-completeness in the study of computational complexity. There is also an introductory treatment of the methods that have been used to deal with *NP*-completeness. We will see a discussion of some of the proposed heuristics in the discussion on the applications of Hopfield nets to the *NP*-complete traveling salesman problem in Chapter 6.

Back-propagation techniques have also been used by Qian (1988) to train a network to predict the secondary structure of a local sequence of amino acids. The input to the trained network are the twenty amino acids and a spacer symbol for regions between proteins, and the output is one of three types of secondary structures: α-helix, β-sheet, and coil. The network was trained using the Brookhaven databank of protein structures.

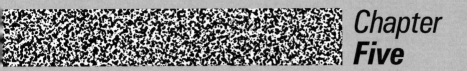

Chapter
Five

Some Learning Paradigms

■ 5.1 Introduction

This chapter is devoted primarily to a discussion of some of the major models that have dominated the literature in the field in recent years — specifically, it presents concise discussions of the competitive learning, interactive activation, and adaptive resonance paradigms. The relationships between these models is explored in the course of the descriptions leading from one to the other. Just as Chapters 2 and 3 have focused on supervised learning, as evidenced by associative memory, so the focus in this chapter is on unsupervised learning; in fact, all three models discussed here execute their learning processes in the absence of supervision. We first present the competitive learning and the interactive activation paradigms and examine their fundamental points of difference. Then the focus shifts to the adaptive resonance paradigm, an attempt to eliminate some of the temporal instabilities of competitive learning. The learning-by-back-propagation model was already introduced in Chapter 4. This chapter shows, in some detail, how it relates to the adaptive resonance paradigm.

It is instructive to pause and reflect on the overabundance of network models that mirror several researchers' intuitions regarding the functioning of the brain. Two models that have different mechanistic rules may have the same collective emergent functional properties. It is this relationship between the emergent properties responsible for determining behavioral success and the mechanisms that generate these properties that is still somewhat unclear. Now, these emergent properties are often more complex than the underlying network components and it becomes essential to employ mathematics that can analyse nonlinear interactions across millions of components, particularly because the emergent properties are not static in the face of learning strategies. Grossberg (1987a) touches on a matter of utmost importance when he points out that it is essential to go beyond the mechanistic details of network models to the deeper architectural level to really understand their relationships to one another.

■ 5.2 The Competitive Learning Paradigm

Competitive learning is an essentially nonassociative statistical learning scheme. Rumelhart (1985) shows how simple adaptive networks can discover features important in the description of the system's stimulus environment. Features discovered in the first layer can be used in the subsequent layers (of a multilayered system) to classify pattern sets that could not easily be classified by a single-layer system. An in-depth consideration of the competitive learning paradigm follows. Many of the properties and architectural details mentioned in the first two sections assume significance in the study of the Linsker and Fukushima models described later.

To understand competitive learning thoroughly, it is necessary to review some of Rosenblatt's related work on *spontaneous learning*. All network learning models require rules, which tell how to present the stimuli and change the values of the weights in accordance with the response of the model. At one end of the spectrum of these rules is learning with an error-correcting teacher, at the other end is completely spontaneous, unsupervised discovery. *Forced learning* refers to the intermediate continuum of rules based on the manipulation of the content of the input stimulus stream to bring about learning. Competitive learning comes under the no-teacher category.

One of Rosenblatt's earlier attempts was to produce a perceptron that would dichotomize patterns into those that produced a 1 response, and those that produced a 0 response, from a net. Weights of lines active with patterns in the 1 set were incremented; those active with patterns in the 0 set were decremented. The fact that weights were allowed to grow without limit implied that the set that had the initial majority of the patterns would receive the majority of the reinforcement and sooner or later all the patterns would end up being classified under one set. To make a dichotomy of patterns a stable state, the rules were modified so that the magnitude of all weights were lowered by a fixed fraction of their current value before specifically incrementing the magnitude of some of the weights on the basis of the response to an input pattern. Rosenblatt claimed that such a perceptron, exemplifying the principle of *statistical separability*, came the closest to approximating the nervous system.

Rosenblatt's result that a two-layer perceptron could carry out any of the 2^{2N} possible classifications of N binary inputs was of little practical value because 2^N units were required to accomplish the task in the general case. Problems of scale appear to exist not only in serial pattern recognizers, but also in parallel recognizing elements. Neural networks are architecturally very sensitive (i.e., small changes in, for instance, node layout can produce significant changes in function). This suggests that creating a general purpose neural net is no easy task. Indeed, the enterprise of creating a network to perform a specific task is very much in the experimental stages. No network is capable of learning what it cannot do in principle and this latter capability depends on the structure and computational properties of its component elements.

5.2.1 The Place of Competitive Learning Among Other Learning Paradigms

Rumelhart (1985) has classified network models on the basis of their learning paradigms.

1. *Auto Associator:* A degraded version of the original pattern can act as a retrieval cue.

2. *Pattern Associator:* A set of pairs of patterns are repeatedly presented. System learns that when one member of the pair is presented, the other is to be brought up.

3. *Classification Paradigm:* A collection of stimulus patterns and their categories are presented. The system learns to respond to a stimulus, distorted or otherwise, with the correct category.

4. *Regularity Detector:* Each stimulus pattern is presented with some probability. System discovers statistically salient features of the input population. There is no a priori set of categories into which the patterns are to be classified; the system develops its own featural representation of the input stimuli.

Competitive learning falls in the last of these categories.

5.2.2 Architectural Framework[1]

Rumelhart (1985) describes the architectural framework of a system employing competitive learning (Fig. 5.1) as one consisting of a set of hierarchically layered units in which each layer connects, via excitatory connections, with the layer immediately above it. Within a layer, the units are broken into a set of nonoverlapping inhibitory clusters in which all elements within a cluster inhibit all other elements in the cluster. Every element in a cluster receives inputs from the same lines from lower layers. A unit learns if and only if it wins the competition with other units in its cluster. Thus the elements within a cluster compete with one another to respond to the pattern appearing on the layer below.

[1]Math in Section 5.2.2 from Rumelhart, D. E., and Zipser, D. (1985). "Feature Discovery by Competitive Learning," *Cognitive Science,* 9(1), 75–112. Reprinted with permission of Ablex Publishing Corporation.

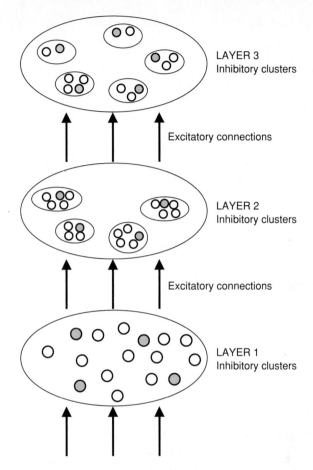

Figure 5.1 *The architecture of the competitive learning mechanism.*

The hierarchically layered units, active (*filled dots*) or inactive (*open dots*), are represented in the diagram as dots. A unit in a given layer can receive inputs from all of the units in the next lower layer and can project outputs to all of the units in the next higher layer. Interlayer connections are excitatory, intralayer ones are inhibitory. Each layer consists of a set of clusters of mutually inhibitory units. Intracluster units inhibit each other so that only one unit may be active at a time. The configuration of active units on any given layer represents the input pattern for the next higher level.

From Rumelhart, David, and Zipser, David, "Feature Discovery by Competitive Learning," Cognitive Science 9, 75–112, 1985. Reprinted with permission.

Since the clusters are winner-take-all, the winning unit is pushed to its maximum value, while all others are forced to their minimum value. The winning unit learns by shifting weight from its inactive to its active input lines (active lines are those connected to the active, that is, in the 1 set, elements of the binary-valued input patterns).

ω_{ij} = weight of line connecting unit i on lower layer to unit j on upper layer,

$$\sum_i \omega_{ij} = 1.$$

Each of the input lines to the winning unit gives up some proportion g of its weight and that weight is then distributed equally among the active input lines, that is,

$$\Delta\omega_{ij} = \begin{cases} 0 & \text{if unit } j \text{ loses on stimulus } k \\ g\dfrac{c_{ik}}{n_k} - g\omega_{ij} & \text{if unit } j \text{ wins on stimulus } k, \end{cases}$$

where

$$c_{ik} = 1$$

if in pattern S_k unit i in the lower layer is active, and 0 otherwise, and

$$n_k = \sum_i c_{ik} = \text{number of active units in pattern } S_k.$$

There is a convenient geometric interpretation given by Rumelhart (1985). If each stimulus pattern is considered to be an N-dimensional vector, then each pattern may be represented by a point on an N-dimensional sphere. The weights of the connections to the units in the upper layer can also be viewed as an N-dimensional vector (since every unit in the upper layer receives N inputs). These, therefore, also lie on the same sphere. The unit that responds most strongly to a stimulus is the one whose weight vector is closest to the stimulus pattern. It does so by moving a percentage g of the way from its current location toward the location of the stimulus pattern on the sphere.

Thus we find that each cluster deals with a separate feature of the input pattern. (The model as described doesn't assure that the different clusters will discover different features. A slight modification of the system in which clusters "repel" one another would be required.) If a cluster has M units in it, we can say that the cluster forms an M-ary feature in which every stimulus pattern is classified as having exactly one of the M possible values of this feature.

The more highly structured the stimuli are, the more stable are the classifications. The grouping done by a particular cluster depends on the starting value of the weights and the sequence of stimulus patterns actually presented.

■ 5.3 The Linsker Model: An Example of Competitive Learning

Linsker (1988) provides an example of feature discovery by competitive learning. His example is motivated by the properties found in the cells of the first few processing stages of the mammalian visual system. Since these properties develop before birth in some animals, they are not the result of any structured experience. The corresponding properties in his network are the result of only random signalling in the network's input layer.

Visual mechanisms provide an appropriate example of feature detection. Simple aspects of form, such as contrast and edge orientation, are analyzed in the earlier layers; these are combined to form more complex features in later layers. Within any retinal or cortical layer, we find groups of cells performing the same function. Each cell processes input from its receptive field, a limited visual space region. Even though a cell's response function is normally nonlinear, a linear summation approximation is appropriate as feature formation occurs in this case too.

In the Linsker model, external input arrives in layer *A*. The cells are organized into two-dimensional layers, *A*, *B*, *C*, and so on with feedforward connections to each cell from an overlying neighborhood of cells of the previous layer (Fig. 5.2). For simplicity, we assume that the intercell connections are fixed. These connections are chosen according to, say, a Gaussian distribution so that a cell has most of its connections in nearby positions in the neighboring layer.

5.3.1 Mathematical Modeling[2]

Let the cells $L_1, L_2, \ldots, L_N$ provide inputs to the cell M. A set of activity values, denoted by $(L_1^\pi, L_2^\pi, \ldots, L_N^\pi)$ is presented to the M cell, which generates an output activity value M^π. The linear response rule is

$$M^\pi = a_1 + \sum_j L_j^\pi c_j,$$

[2]Math in Section 5.3.1 from Linsker, "Self-Organization in a Perceptual Network," *Computer*, March 1988, 105–117. © 1988 IEEE. Reprinted with permission.

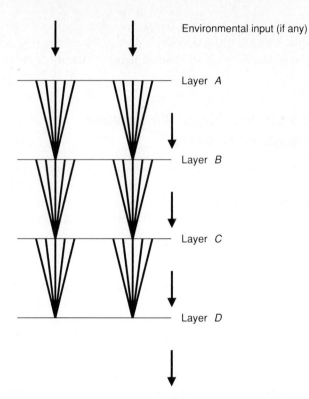

Environmental input (if any)

Layer *A*

Layer *B*

Layer *C*

Layer *D*

Figure 5.2 *A layered self-adaptive network with local feedforward connection.*

where

$\qquad c_j$ = strength of the jth input connection to the M cell.

Here, the superscript π is merely an identifier for a snapshot in the system's development. This model uses the following variation of the Hebb rule

$$(\Delta c_i)^\pi = a_2 L_i^\pi M^\pi + a_3 L_i^\pi + a_4 M^\pi + a_5,$$

where the only constraint on the constants is that $a_2 > 0$ (Hebb rule).

If this result is averaged over an ensemble of several presentations and the earlier expression for M^π is used, after some algebraic manipulation we have

$$\frac{dc_i}{dt} = \sum_j Q_{ij} c_j + \left[k_1 + \left(\frac{k_2}{N}\right) \sum c_j \right],$$

where

$k_{1,2}$ = particular combinations of the constants a_{1-5} and

$$Q_{ij} = \langle (L_i^\pi - \bar{L}) \times (L_j^\pi - \bar{L}) \rangle.$$

Here Q_{ij} is the covariance of the activities of input cells i and j (a particular entry of this matrix may be nonzero even if the corresponding neurons are not directly linked together because of the way in which the modified Hebbian rule is defined) and the operator $\langle \cdot \cdot \rangle$ denotes the ensemble average (i.e., expectation). Also $\bar{L}$ is the ensemble average of the input activity at a synapse and is assumed to be the same for all the synapses. Note also that to prevent saturation, each c value is presumed to lie between two values c_- and c_+.

The computation of the connection strengths for successive layers is recursive. Using the Q_{ij} matrix for input layer A, the connection strengths for the A-to-B layer are computed. Then, using these values and the Q_{ij} matrix for B, the connection strengths for the B-to-C layer are computed, and so on. Linsker (1988) shows that there is a limited number of ways that a layer can develop as there are only a few parameters that determine the mature c values of cells. These parameters include $k_{1,2}$ and the size of the receptive field of the cells in the developing layer.

New cell types emerge in the layers in this fashion. If the input to A was random, then *center-surround* cell types, acting as *contrast-sensitive filters* (which respond maximally to either a bright circular spot centered on a dark background or a dark spot on a bright background), emerge in layer C. Further, *orientation-selective cells* (which respond maximally to a bright edge against a dark background, or the reverse, when the bar has a particular orientation) emerge in layer D. By judicious introduction of lateral inhibitory connections, the orientations to which the D-layer cells respond to can be controlled. Thus, a series of progressively more complex feature-analyzing cell types emerge in successive layers.

It is instructive to consider a statistical justification for the Hebbian rule. The assumption in the above model of the ensemble statistical properties of the L-cell activities not depending on the choice of c values is true if there is no feedback from M, or the cells it influences, to the L cells. Define the function E to be

$$E \equiv E_Q + E_k,$$

where

$$E_Q \equiv -\frac{1}{2}\langle(M^\pi - \overline{M})^2\rangle$$

$$= -\frac{1}{2}\sum_i \sum_j Q_{ij}c_ic_j$$

and

$$E_k \equiv -k_1\sum_j c_j - \left(\frac{k_2}{2N}\right)\left(\sum c_j\right)^2.$$

This satisfies

$$-\frac{\partial E}{\partial c_i} = c_i \qquad \forall\, i.$$

As the c values change with time, E (as a function of c's) decreases along a path of locally steepest, or gradient, descent. The value of E thus achieves a local minimum at cell maturity; this, for the two kinds of feature detecting cells mentioned above, is almost a global-minimum as well. Clearly, E is minimized when the statistical variance of M's activity is maximized, that is, when $\langle(M^\pi - \overline{M})\rangle$ is maximized.

Therefore, the cell develops to maximize the variance of its output activity, subject to the constraint that the total of the connection strengths have a given, parameter-determined value and subject to the saturation bounds for each c value. If, as an extreme case, the output of the cell remained constant (zero variance), then the cell would relay no information. At the other extreme, maximizing variance implies ability to convey maximal information. Therefore, the output activity optimally preserves the information contained in the set of input activities.

Linsker (1988) demonstrates how this network can be used for associative retrieval. If few memory patterns are to be stored then the local minima of the E_Q function will be at those $\{c_i\}$ corresponding to those memories. The memory state that is activated depends on the initial state of the c connections. *Selected* means that the final set of c values will cause the M cell to be a *matched filter* for one of these memories. The ability of the E_Q function to capture details of the patterns decreases as the number of patterns increases. As this number increases, the mature M cell becomes a feature-analyzing cell rather than a matched filter to a particular memory. It is perfectly conceivable that the actual feature responded to need not even appear in any of the presented patterns.

In the special case where the sum of the squares of the c values is unity, variance maximization is achieved with the following (equivalent) form of the Hebbian rule,

$$\dot{c}_i \propto \langle M^\pi (L_i^\pi - M^\pi c_i) \rangle.$$

Here, $M^\pi = \Sigma L_i \pi c_i$ and the activities are defined so that $\langle L_i^\pi \rangle = 0$ for all i.

5.3.2 Principal Component Analysis

Principal component analysis (PCA), is a method for identifying interesting but unanticipated structure (e.g., clustering) in high-dimensional data sets (Fig. 5.3). Consider a set of data points L^π having coordinates $(L_1^\pi, L_2^\pi, \ldots, L_N^\pi)$. For PCA, we compute a vector c for which the projection of the set of data points onto the axis parallel to c has maximum variance.

The projection of L^π onto c is just

$$M^\pi = \sum_i L_i^\pi c_i$$

when

$$\sum_i c_i^2 = 1,$$

and therefore the variance of this projected distribution is the same as that of M^π. Since the PCA method corresponds to choosing c so as to maximize the variance of M^π, the Hebbian rule stated above performs PCA on its set of inputs.

Now, it turns out that the conditions that c needs to satisfy to perform PCA on their inputs are the same required for the satisfaction of the *principle of optimal inference*. This is stated briefly as follows. Suppose

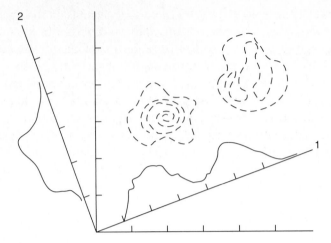

Figure 5.3 *Illustration of principal component analysis.*

The density plots formed by projecting the cloud of data points onto each of two axes are shown. Projection onto axis 1 has maximum variance and clearly shows the bimodal or clustered character of the data.

that we know the c values, and are told a particular value of the output, M^{π}. We are asked to estimate the input activities $(L_1^{\pi}, L_2^{\pi}, \ldots, L_N^{\pi})$ and the quality of our estimation is gauged by computing the mean square error (MSE):

$$\text{MSE} = \sum_i \langle [L_i^{\pi} - L_i^{\pi}(\text{est})]^2 \rangle,$$

where

$$L_i^{\pi} = \text{true values and}$$
$$L_i^{\pi}(\text{est}) = \text{estimated values.}$$

The optimal inference of the input activity values occurs when MSE is minimized.

Linsker (1988) points out that such results suggest that, at least in an intuitive way, a Hebbian rule may act to generate an M cell whose output activity *preserves maximum information* about the input activities, subject to constraints. It turns out that the idea of maximal preservation applies to the development of each layer of a competitive learning perceptual system. Some background to understand this principle, also called the *infomax principle,* is provided below.

5.3.3 Shannon Information and the Infomax Principle[3]

Each presentation of $L = (L_1, L_2, \ldots, L_N)$ is a message where L_i denotes the activity of the ith L cell in the layer. Think of the N-dimensional space of the L vectors as being divided into small boxes, each labeled by its location L. Two messages are regarded as identical if they lie in the same box. Further, let $P(L)$ be the probability that a message lies in box L. If $I(L)$ denotes the information in a message, then

$$I(L) = -\ln P(L).$$

Average information per message is

$$\langle [-\ln P(L)] \rangle = -\sum_L P(L) \ln P(L).$$

If we are told which discrete box the vector M lies in, then the amount of additional information that we need to reconstruct the input message L that gave rise to M is given by

$$I_M(L) = \left[-\ln P\left(\frac{L}{M}\right) \right]$$

where

$$P\left(\frac{L}{M}\right) = \text{conditional probability that input is in box } L \text{ given that output is in box } M.$$

It follows that the amount of information that knowing M tells us about L is

$$I(L) - I_M(L) = \ln\left[\frac{P(L/M)}{P(L)}\right],$$

and the average of this quantity is the rate per message R of transmission of information from the cell's inputs to its output:

$$R = \left\langle \ln\left[\frac{P(L/M)}{P(L)}\right]\right\rangle,$$

Using the simple probabilistic identity, $P(L/M) \cdot P(M) = P(L \cdot M) = P(M/L) \cdot P(L)$, R can be rewritten as

$$R = \left\langle \ln\left[\frac{P(M/L)}{P(M)}\right]\right\rangle,$$

$$\Rightarrow R = -\langle \ln P(M)\rangle + \left\langle \ln P\left(\frac{M}{L}\right)\right\rangle, \quad \text{and}$$

$$\Rightarrow R = \langle I(M)\rangle - \langle I_L(M)\rangle.$$

This is the average of the total information conveyed by M, minus the information that M conveys to one who already knows L. Therefore, $\langle I_L(M)\rangle$ is the information that M conveys about processing noise rather than about the signal L.

If cell layer L is to provide inputs to another cell layer M, then the manner in which such inputs are transferred is such that the rate R of (Shannon) information transmission from L to M is maximized. This is the statement of the infomax principle.

To relate this to the maximal variance results for single cells, Linsker (1988) derives (under reasonable assumptions) an expression for the rate of information in a single cell to be

$$R = \frac{1}{2}\ln\left(\frac{V}{B}\right),$$

where

    V = output variance of the cell and
    B = noise variance.

When B is fixed, maximizing Shannon information corresponds to maximizing output variance.

Consider a system with an arbitrary number of L cells and only two coupled M cells,

$$M_j^\pi = \left(\sum_i t_{ji} L_i^\pi \right) + v_j^\pi \qquad \text{for } j = 1, 2 .$$

Under standard assumptions, R is calculated to be

$$R = \frac{1}{2} \ln(\text{Det } Q^M) - \ln B,$$

where Q^M is a 2×2 covariance matrix such that

$$Q_{nm}^M = \langle M_n^\pi M_m^\pi \rangle$$

and

$$\text{Det } Q^M = B^2 + B(W_1 + W_2) + W_1 W_2 (1 - \rho_{12}^2)$$

Here

W_k is the output variance of cell M_k and
ρ_{12} is the correlation coefficient of cell output activities.

Maximizing R implies maximizing Det Q^M. When there is a high-noise level (large B), maximizing Det Q^M implies maximizing the sum of the W's. This can be achieved if each cell maximizes its output variance separately. If there is only one input combination that yields maximal output variance, both cells will compute it independently. Therefore, a high-noise level favors redundancy, as this mitigates the information-destroying effects of noise. In contrast, a low-noise level (small B) implies that Det Q^M is maximized by making an optimal tradeoff between keeping the W's large and making the responses of the two M cells uncorrelated. A lower-noise level favors diversity of response as the informational value of the cells extracting different input combinations outweighs the resulting disadvantage of each cell's output variance being slightly smaller.

These results do extend to systems having many more than two M cells. If the noise variance B is large and if few M cells "see" the same set of L cells, we expect to see the M cells developing so as to maximize individual activity variance and thereby instituting redundancy to counteract the high-noise level. In contrast, if B is small and many M cells see the same L region, then the M cells do not perform the same processing function on the L layer inputs. They may, in fact, span a range of feature-analyzing properties.

The infomax dictum that the information that reaches a layer is processed so that the maximum amount is preserved does not, in general, imply a one-to-one mapping in which each M cell receives input from only one L cell. Noise prevents the identity mapping from maximally preserving information. Instead, each cell responds to statistically and information-theoretically significant features, much in the way that principal component analysis operates. An analogy drawn from management is illustrative. In some sense, the cells in various layers correspond to the bureaucrats of varying stature. The lowest-level cells simply collate information, and as one moves higher each level summarises information received from previous levels. The complexity of the summary increases as one rises in the hierarchy. Since the low-level workers do not need to know what the overall goals of the organization are and the superior management cells do not need the insignificant data filtered out by the lower levels, local optimization principles can be employed.

■ 5.4 The Fukushima Models: Another Example of Competitive Learning

Fukushima (1975) also employs competitive learning in his multilayered neural network called the *cognitron*. The cognitron was developed in response to the observation that the neural nets in the visual centers of the brain developed so as to recognize features in the input patterns presented to them.

5.4.1 Implications of a Modified Hebbian Rule

An augmented Hebbian rule is used here and can be stated as follows:

The synaptic connection from cell x to cell y is reinforced if and only if the following two conditions are simultaneously satisfied: (1) presynaptic cell x fires and (2) none of the postsynaptic cells situated near the cell y fires more strongly than y.

The region from which a cell can have its afferent (input) synapses is called its *connectable area*, while the region to which its efferent (output) synapses connect is called the *vicinity area*. Plasticity implies that all synapses in the connectable area need not exist simultaneously. Condition 2 suggests that the cell *y* fires the strongest among all those in its vicinity area. Note that if no vicinity cell fires, all the efferent synapses are strengthened. Under this circumstance, however, the strengthening is less than in the case when at least one vicinity cell does fire. A biological reason justifies this intuitive result. Synaptic strengthening requires a secretion from a glia cell. The spread of one glia cell coincides with a vicinity area. Since there is a limited amount of strengthening material available, it must be distributed to the synapses that need to be strengthened. The more these number, the weaker the strengthening. Further, note that because of Condition 2, any slight difference in characteristics between the cells will grow more and more pronounced. This appears to favour the development of feature-detecting cells. A damaged cell will be substituted for by another cell. When damage causes a cell with a certain characteristic to cease to respond, its place is taken by the cell with the next strongest response to that characteristic. This then grows stronger. Thus, a *self-repairing* function is instituted.

5.4.2 The Cognitron

The neural element in the Fukushima cognitron assumes nonnegative analog output values given by

$$
w = \phi\left[\frac{1 + \sum_{\nu=1}^{N} a(\nu) \cdot u(\nu)}{1 + \sum_{\mu=1}^{M} b(\mu) \cdot v(\mu)} - 1\right],
$$

where

$$
\phi[x] = \begin{cases} x & (x \geq 0) \\ 0 & (x < 0). \end{cases}
$$

Here $u(1), u(2), \ldots, u(N)$ are the inputs from the excitatory afferent synapses and $v(1), v(2), \ldots, v(M)$ are the inputs from the inhibitory afferent synapses. Also,

$a(\nu)$ = nonnegative analog conductances of the excitatory synapses and

$b(\mu)$ = nonnegative analog conductances of the inhibitory synapses.

Further, if e and h are the sum of the excitatory and inhibitory effects, respectively, that is,

$$e = \sum_{\nu=1}^{N} a(\nu) \cdot u(\nu)$$

$$h = \sum_{\mu=1}^{M} b(\mu) \cdot v(\mu)$$

then, we can rewrite the expression for the output as

$$w = \phi\left[\frac{1 + e}{1 + h} - 1\right] = \phi\left[\frac{e - h}{1 + h}\right].$$

Note that, for a cognitron-like system where the synapses are being continually strengthened, we cannot have analog-threshold elements because of saturation problems. Since, for small h, the above expression is essentially $w = (e - h)$, this is inappropriate. However, if both $e \gg 1$ and $h \gg 1$, then $w = (e/h - 1)$ and the cell output converges to a certain value so long as both the excitatory and the inhibitory synaptic conductances increase with the same rate.

Neural elements satisfying these properties form the many layers of the cognitron. The excitatory cells within any layer l receive inputs of two kinds—that is, excitatory inputs from excitatory cells in the previous $(l - 1)$th layer and inhibitory inputs from inhibitory cells in the $(l - 1)$th layer. Further, the inhibitory cells in the $(l - 1)$th layer receive inputs from the excitatory cells in the same $(l - 1)$th layer (i.e., the connectable area of an excitatory cell is the same as that of an inhibitory cell in the previous layer) and output the average of these values to the excitatory cell in the lth layer. This setup recursively defines the cognitron's structure (see Fig. 5.4).

Fukushima's (1975) results basically ratify the competitive learning precepts. Excitatory connections are more reinforced than inhibitory ones when the cell displays a high output; conversely, inhibitory connections are more reinforced (i.e., made more inhibitory) when the cell has a low output. Further, the cognitron's ability to differentiate a pattern from other similar ones arises as a result of the strong reinforcement of inhibitory connections (when a cell has low output), which makes postsynaptic cells reluctant to respond to stimulus patterns other than the one to which the cell has been reinforced.

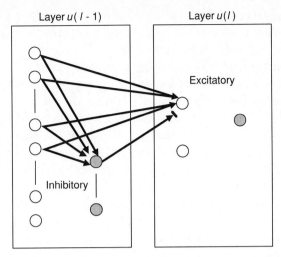

Layer $u(l-1)$

Layer $u(l)$

Excitatory

Inhibitory

Figure 5.4 *Two adjacent layers of the cognitron.*

This figure shows that the connectable area of an excitatory cell is the same as that of an inhibitory cell in the previous layer.

From Fukushima, Kunihiko, "Cognitron: A Self-Organizing Multilayered Neural Network," Biological Cybernetics 20, 121–136, 1975. Reprinted with permission.

5.4.3 The Neocognitron[4]

Fukushima (1980) modifies the cognitron to get around its primary flaw (i.e., the response of the cognitron was severely affected by the shift in position and/or by the distortion in shape of the input patterns, thus limiting its use as a pattern recognition device). In the resulting augmented hierarchical model called the *neocognitron*, the cells in the highest stages are supposed to respond, in a position-invariant manner, to specific stimulus patterns.

In the neocognitron, we see stacked modular structures each composed of two cascaded layers containing (1) *S*-cells corresponding to simple cells and (2) *C*-cells corresponding to complex cells. Only the input synapses to *S*-cells are supposed to have plasticity and be modifiable. Within each layer (*S* or *C*) some cells are grouped together to form cell planes. Since all cells in a single cell plane have input synapses of the same spatial distribution, their receptive fields are functionally equiva-

---

[4]From Fukushima, "Neocognitron: Self-Organizing Neural Network Model for Mechanism of Pattern Recognition Unaffected by Shift in Position," *Biological Cybernetics*, 36, 193–202. © 1980. Springer/Verlag. Reprinted with permission.

lent. However, the positions of the presynaptic cells may vary for each cell in a given cell field. Therefore, the receptive fields of cells in a cell field will occur at different positions.

The learning procedure is roughly as follows. As with all competitive learning systems, the process is unsupervised. Initially, the modifiable synapses are set to have small positive values so that the S-cells show very weak orientation selectivity, and the preferred orientation of the S-cells differ from S-plane to S-plane. Imagine all the S-planes within an S-layer being stacked one atop the other to form an S-column. Now, when a stimulus pattern is presented to the S-column, the S-cell yielding the largest output is chosen as a candidate for reenforcement. In all events of at least one maximal response, only one candidate is chosen from each S-plane. Eventually, each S-plane becomes selectively sensitive to some feature in the input pattern. No two S-planes can detect the same feature.

Thus, a number of feature-extracting cells of the same function are formed in parallel within each S-plane, and only the positions of their receptive fields differ. Indeed, this is the basis of the position invariance of the neocognitron. If a stimulus pattern that elicits a response from an S-cell is shifted, another S-cell in the same S-plane will respond to it. Since the C-cell responds strongly whenever at least one S-cell in its connecting area yields a large output, shifting of the stimulus pattern will not effect the C-cell's response. There is a simple way to relate the cognitron with its augmented model, the neocognitron. If a single S-plane in the latter corresponds to a single excitatory cell in the cognitron, the procedures of reenforcement are seen to be largely similar in both systems.

■ *5.5 The Interactive Activation Paradigm*[5]

The interactive activation model is proposed as one capable of explaining the fundamental facts of word perception. The most simplistic version limits the processing to just three hierarchical levels, the feature, letter, and word levels. The basis of this model is as follows: A visual input excites detectors for visual features in the display. These excite detectors of letters consistent with the active features. These in turn excite detectors for consistent words. Active word detectors mutually inhibit each other

[5]From McClelland, "Interactive Activation Model of Context Effects in Letter Perception: Part 1: An Account of Basic Findings," *Psychological Review,* 88, No. 5, 375–407. © 1981 by the American Psychological Association. Adapted by permission of the publisher.

and send feedback to the letter level, strengthening activation and hence perceptibility of their constituent letters.

McClelland (1981) states that until recently it has been possible to imagine that the context in which a letter was presented influences only the accuracy of postperceptual processes and not the process of perception itself. However, Reicher's (1969) findings have indicated that subjects actually come away with more information relevant to a choice between the alternatives when the target letter is a part of a word. Letters in words are more perceptible because they receive more activation than representations of either single letters or letters in an unrelated context. Some other results related to word-advantage are: the effect is independent of the familiarity of the word as a visual configuration (word shape); the advantage is enhanced when the target appears in a distinct high-contrast display; the advantage also applies to pronounceable nonwords, for example, reet or mave; letters in highly constraining word contexts have little or no advantage over letters in weakly constraining word contexts.

Salient assumptions of the *interactive activation model* (Fig. 5.5) are as follows:

1. Each of the several levels of processing are concerned with forming a representation of the input at a different level of abstraction.

2. Two kinds of parallelisms are inherent in the model. Spatial parallelism arises from the capability to process several letters of a word at one time. In addition processes operate simultaneously at several different levels.

3. Perception is an interactive process. Top-down, or conceptually driven, processing works in conjunction with bottom-up, or data driven, processing to provide a multiplicity of constraints that jointly determine perception.

4. The model of interaction uses simple excitatory and inhibitory activations of a neural type.

Communication, consisting of both excitatory and inhibitory messages, proceeds through a spreading activation mechanism in which activation at one level spreads to neighboring levels and alters the activation level of the recipient(s). Connections may occur within levels or between adjacent levels; never between nonadjacent levels. Intralevel inhibitory loops represent a kind of lateral inhibition in which incompatible units

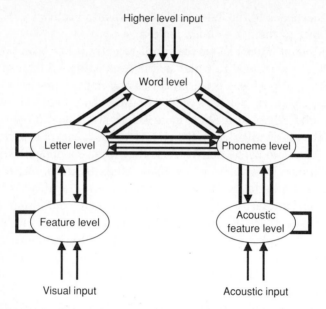

Figure 5.5 *Use the interactive activation model in visual and auditory word perception.*

From McClelland, "Interactive Activation Model of Context Effects in Letter Perception: Part1: An Account of Basic Findings," Psychological Review, 58, No.5, 375–407. Copyright ©1981 by the American Psychological Association. Reprinted by permission of the publisher.

at the same level compete. Interlevel connections may be either excitatory or inhibitory.

A node is active if its activation value is positive. In the absence of inputs, nodes decay to an inactive state (i.e., to an activation value at or below zero):

$a_i(t)$ = activation value for node i at time t,

r_i = resting level for node i ($r_i \propto$ frequency of occurence of word), and

$\theta_i(t)$ = rate at which decay to the resting level occurs.

If $n_i(t)$ represents the net input to unit i, then

$$n_i(t) = \sum_j \alpha_{ij} e_j(t) - \sum_k \gamma_{ik} i_k(t),$$

where

$e_j(t)$ = activation of an active excitatory neighbor of node i,
$i_k(t)$ = activation of an active inhibitory neighbor of node i, and
α_{ij}, γ_{ik} are associated weight constants.

The degree of the effect of the input on the node is modulated by the node's current activity level to keep the input to the node from driving it beyond some maximum and minimum limits.

For net excitation, if $\varepsilon_i(t)$ is the effect on the node

$$\varepsilon_i(t) = n_i(t)(M - a_i(t)),$$

where

M = maximum activation level of the unit.

Similarly, for net inhibition

$$\varepsilon_i(t) = n_i(t)(a_i(t) - m),$$

where

m = minimum activation of the unit.

Taking into account the decaying of the node, the new activation is given by

$$a_i(t + \Delta t) = a_i(t) - \theta_i(a_i(t) - r_i) + \varepsilon_i(t).$$

Inputs to the network present a set of binary (i.e., either present or absent) features, each of which will be detected (it is assumed that detection is instantaneous) with probability p. Letter level nodes that do not contain the extracted feature are inhibited. Presentation of a new display following an old one results in the probabilistic extraction of the set of features present in the new display.

It is assumed that responses and perhaps the contents of perceptual experience depend on the temporal integration of the activation pattern over all of the nodes. Specifically, the integration process takes a running average of the node activation over previous time:

$$\bar{a}_i(t) = \int_{-\infty}^{t} a_i(x)e^{-(t-x)r} dx,$$

where

    r = relative weighting given to old and new information.

Response strength is an exponential function of the running average activation:

$$s_i(t) = e^{\mu \bar{a}_i(t)}.$$

The probability of making a response based on node i is given by

$$p(R_i, t) = \frac{s_i(t)}{\sum\limits_{j \in L} s_j(t)},$$

where L represents the set of nodes competing at the same level with i.

When the target display is simply turned on and left on until the subject responds, and there is no pressure to respond quickly, it is assumed that the subject waits until the output strengths have reached their asymptotic values. If a target display is presented briefly followed by a patterned mask, the activations produced by the target are transient.

The interactive activation model described above can be considered to be a relaxation scheme that attempts to optimally interpret an input word by manipulating the activation levels of its hidden units. While earlier models advocated a similar hierarchical approach to processing of input, the interesting part of this model is the manner in which processing at all levels of the hierarchy occurs in parallel. Partial outputs are continuously available for processing at each stage and information flows in both directions simultaneously.

Consider the simple task of reading. The perception of any individual letter occurs during the simultaneous perception of the several other letters around it that serve to create its context. Rumelhart (1982) conducted a series of experiments to demonstrate the temporal course of the facilitation that context provides for the perception of target letters. For instance, it is shown that the duration and timing of the presentation of the contextual information greatly influences the perception of the target letter. Some of the experiments performed include determining whether the perceptibility of a letter in a word depends on the duration of the context letters in the display, showing that the arrival of contextual information early primes the node of the target and facilitates target perception while presentation of the context following that of the target is of little use, and examining the relative importance of additional contextual information versus additional direct evidence.

The conclusions that these experiments with the interactive activation model have resulted in are as follows. Quite simply, the longer the duration of the context and the larger the number of context letters enhanced, the more accurate was forced-choice performance on the target letter. That the context clearly affects perception is confirmed by the fact that letters in nonwords that are similar to words are far easier to perceive than are letters embedded in, for instance, a host of numerals or in an ensemble of letters grouped together in a manner not consistent with the statistical regularities of English letter strings.

■ 5.6 Comparison of the Competitive Learning and Interactive Activation Paradigms

Grossberg (1987a) points out that both the levels and the interactions of these two paradigms are incompatible. The first major point of difference is that the interlevel interactions that are found in the interactive activation model cannot be reproduced in the competitive learning paradigm. In competitive learning, all interlevel connections are excitatory whereas in interactive activation, interlevel connections are selectively excitatory or inhibitory. This selectiveness is something that has to be learned, and Grossberg (1987a) shows that such learning cannot occur in the competitive learning model.

The second point of difference is that the letter level and the word level of the interactive activation model do not exist in a language learning model based upon competitive learning. To appreciate this, consider the argument postulated by Grossberg (1987a). McClelland (1981) requires that a stage of letter nodes precede the processing of letters appearing as words in the next layer. Though McClelland (1981) uses the specific example of four-letter words in the word layer, their interactive activation concept should generalize to words of any length, in particular single-letter words. This implies that those letters that are also words (e.g., "A" and "I") would appear on both the letter and the word layers, whereas letters that are not words in and of themselves would only appear in the letter layer. This distinction could not be learned by an unsupervised learning scheme like competitive learning.

Further, Grossberg (1987a) asks the following questions of the interactive activation model. What did the nodes representing particular letters (or words) represent before these letters (or words) were learned? Also, where will the nodes come from to represent letters (or words) that have not yet been learned? The fact that single-letter words exist separately in the letter and word levels suggests that these levels should be able to enforce each other and result in it being easier to recognize single-letter words than other words. Grossberg (1987a) points out that other literature shows that this is not the case.

■ 5.7 Adaptive Resonance Theory: A Stabilized Version of Competitive Learning[5]

Thus far, we have introduced the competitive learning and the interactive activation paradigms. These paradigms, and others that learn in an unsupervised fashion, represent attempts to fulfill one of computer science's main goals — that of developing an intelligent machine that can perform satisfactorily in an unaided fashion in a complex environment. Unfortunately, certain stability problems preclude the satisfaction of this goal by any of these paradigms. The remainder of this chapter discusses the adaptive learning paradigm, an attempt to endow the competitive learning paradigm with stability. Finally, we discuss how this paradigm relates to the back-propagation paradigm. The back-propagation paradigm, also referred to as the generalized delta rule, has already been discussed in some detail in Chapter 4.

In has been proved that, in certain input environments, if the number of patterns presented to the input layer of a competitive learning system is not too large relative to the number of coding nodes in the output layer, then the learned recognition code stabilizes and the best distribution of long-term memory (LTM) traces, hitherto referred to as adaptive weights, results. However, in arbitrary input environments, competitive learning might not be able to learn a temporally stable code. Thus, repeated presentation of the same stimulus pattern to the system can result in different responses; further, this behavior might never settle as learn-

[5]From Grossberg, S., (1987). "Competitive Learning: From Interactive Activation to Adaptive Resonance," *Cognitive Science*, 11, 23–63. Reprinted with permission of Ablex Publishing Corporation.

ing proceeds. Essentially, each input causes modification to the LTM traces so that subsequent presentations of the same input will be reacted to differently. This is referred to as the *stability-plasticity dilemma.* Grossberg (1987a) describes it thus:

> How can a learning system be designed to remain plastic, or adaptive, in response to significant events and yet remain stable in response to irrelevant events? How does the system know how to switch between its stable and its plastic modes to achieve stability without rigidity and plasticity without chaos? In particular, how can it preserve its previously learned knowledge while continuing to learn new things? What prevents the new learning from washing away the memories of prior learning?

The purpose of the *adaptive resonance theory* (ART) was to show how to embed a competitive learning model into a self-regulating control structure whose autonomous learning and recognition proceeded stably in response to an arbitrary input pattern sequence. In fact, the LTM traces of an ART model oscillate at most once during learning in the face of an arbitrary input sequence.

In addition to having a filter contained in the pathways leading from an initial feature representation field F_1 to a category representation field F_2, as in the competitive learning model, the ART model also has a top-down adaptive filter contained in the pathways leading from F_2 to F_1. It is the existence of these pathways that distinguishes ART from competitive learning architecturally, and it is the self-stabilizing role that these pathways play that distinguishes the two models functionally.

When the nodes of F_1 are activated by an input pattern I, a pattern of activation X is generated across the F_1 nodes. X is said to represent I in short-term memory (STM). This activation is then gated by the weights (LTM traces) in the pathways leading from F_1 to F_2 and generates another activation level, T, across the F_2 nodes. This process is referred to as bottom-up adaptive filtering in Grossberg (1987a). Now, in much the same way that the competitive learning model functions, one of the F_2 nodes, representing a particular category, is selected. This node (category) has its own idea of what activation it represents. Let us call this Y. Grossberg (1987a) refers to this as the contrast-enhanced pattern. We can say that Y represents T in STM. Now, Y generates a pattern of activity U that is gated by the LTM traces in the feedback pathways from F_2 to F_1. This generates the activation pattern V at the F_1 nodes. This process is referred to as top-down template matching and V plays the role of learned expectation. Now, the bottom-up input pattern I, which initiated this whole process, and the top-down pattern V both perturb the nodes of F_1. F_1 tries to match V against I and comes up with a new activity pattern X^*. Note that the entire activation chain $I \rightarrow X \rightarrow S \rightarrow T \rightarrow Y \rightarrow U \rightarrow V \rightarrow X^*$ proceeds very quickly relative to the rate at which the weights (LTM traces) in either the top-down or the bottom-up adaptive filter can change.

The system described above is really only the attentional portion of the ART architecture. It is complemented by the orienting subsystem A, whose function is basically to fire a reset-burst toward the F_2 nodes under certain circumstances (discussed below). The input pattern I also activates A, but the STM trace X inhibits A from firing. Now the amount by which the pattern X is attenuated to generate X^* depends upon how much of I is present within the template pattern V (i.e., the greater the extent of the mismatch, the greater the attenuation). When X is attenuated, its inhibitory impact on the orienting subsystem is diminished. This fires a reset burst toward the F_2 nodes resulting in the removal of the top-down template V and in the termination of the mismatch between V and I at the F_1 nodes. The patterns leading to the activation chain now repeat themselves in order to generate another top-down template against which I can be compared at the F_1 nodes. The template V is prevented from being reselected by the long-term nature of the reset burst fired by the orienting subsystem.

The cycle of bottom-up adaptive filtering from F_1 to F_2, template selection at F_2, communication of the template from F_2 to F_1, matching at F_1, and reset at F_2 repeats itself at a fast rate until one of three possibilities occurs:

1. A template is found that approximately matches the input pattern I.

2. A previously uncommitted F_2 node is found (which will then adopt the pattern I as a template).

3. The system capacity is exhausted and cannot accommodate I.

Modification of the LTM traces (weights) occurs only in the first of these three eventualities. The fused pattern X^* (which results when input I is compared to a sufficiently similar template V), represents the attentional focus of the system. The bottom-up and top-down signal patterns get locked into a resonant state of STM activation. It is then that the LTM traces learn any new information about the input pattern represented within the fused activation pattern across F_1. The term *adaptive resonance theory* reflects the fact that learning occurs only in the resonant state.

The *two-thirds rule,* as described by Grossberg (1987a), is used to govern the interaction between the input pattern and the template pattern at the F_1 node level. Supraliminal activation of F_1 nodes, which occurs in response to an arbitrary bottom-up input pattern, is enough to generate output signals toward other parts of the network. Subliminal activation of F_1 nodes, in response to arbitrary top-down expectations, prepares F_1 nodes for future input patterns that may or may not be approximate matches of the expectation but cannot, by itself, generate an output signal. A third F_1 input source, called an *attentional gain control channel,* is used to distinguish between the top-down and the bottom-up inputs. By the two-thirds rule, supraliminal activation of an F_1 node requires that at least two of the three inputs (bottom-up, top-down, and gain control) to the F_1 node be active. During top-down processing, each F_1 node receives a signal from only one source and so can be only subliminally activated. During bottom-up processing, each active bottom-up pathway can turn on the gain control node (which provides an input to all F_1 nodes). Thus nonactive bottom-up nodes receive inputs only from the gain control node. Active bottom-up nodes, on the other hand, receive inputs from the gain control node and the bottom-up pattern and are supraliminally activated. Finally, when template and input pattern matching is taking place, the gain control is shut off. So only those F_1 nodes that receive confirmation of the bottom-up input are supraliminally activated. Thus it is indeed possible that, in the event of a mismatch, fewer F_1 nodes are active during the pattern matching stage than during the presentation of the input stage. This represents a decrease in activity in F_1, hence a decrease in the inhibitory effect of the F_1 nodes on the orienting subsystem mentioned earlier. Thus a mismatch allows the orienting subsystem to fire a reset burst toward the F_2 nodes.

The amount of mismatch tolerated before a template is rejected as not sufficiently matching the input pattern is determined by the vigilance parameter. An ART system with low vigilance will permit large amounts of mismatch and will result in patterns of activity that are only grossly similar being grouped together. This is in contrast to high-vigilance systems, which try and form separate categories for systems that have only minor differences. The change in vigilance may be interpreted as a change in the system's attentional state that increases its sensitivity to mismatches.

Grossberg (1987a) effectively summarises the above discussion by providing four properties that are deemed essential to an ART network. These are mentioned briefly here.

1. *Recognition of Critical Feature Patterns:* The ART network is able to incorporate the notion of pattern context into its determination of whether a particular input feature is a signal or is merely noise. A particular feature may be a signal in one context and noise in another. Critical feature patterns are the computational units of the code learning process and the learned units are patterns of critical features.

2. *Self-Adjusting Memory Search:* Faced with the possibility of evolving into an arbitrarily complex structure in the face of continual learning, it is not possible to have a predetermined search algorithm that will always be the most efficient. The parallel memory search of an ART system adaptively updates its search order to maintain efficiency.

3. *Direct Access to Learned Codes:* In the ART architecture, as the learned code becomes increasingly predictively accurate, the search mechanism is automatically disengaged. Thus, unambiguous events are rapidly detected. In contrast, the search time in trees and other serial algorithms increases as the learned recognition code becomes increasingly large.

4. *Environment as a Teacher:* Though the ART system represents an unsupervised learning paradigm, the environment can modulate the teaching process by adjusting the vigilance parameter. Thus, if a particular input pattern is taken as matching a particular template, and the environment disapproves, then an external teacher can increase the vigilance parameter and make sure that the erroneous mismatch does not re-occur.

ART models are most suited to learn and respond in real time to a nonstationary world with an unlimited number of inputs until it utilizes its full memory capacity. In supervised (teacher) learning systems, the learning is often driven by mismatch between desired and actual outputs. Interaction with the teacher slows the system down. The external teacher is required not only to provide the desired output for comparison with the actual but also to prevent *capacity catastrophe.* (This occurs in non–self-stabilizing systems when an unlimited input stream results in memories of prior learning being washed away. To prevent this, either the input stream should be curtailed or learning should be shut off. The teacher determines when such preventive action becomes imperative.) Further, in some other learning systems (e.g., simulated annealing and Boltzmann machines), there is the possibility of getting trapped in local minima or in a globally incorrect solution. Since ART relies on approximate matches (rather than mismatches) to further its learning and does so in the absence of external teachers and external controlling factors such as temperature, the process can occur stably while buffering the system's memory against external noise.

■ 5.8 Comparison of the Adaptive Resonance and Learning-by-Back-Propagation Paradigms

The primary difference between the ART and the back-propagation (BP) models is that the former provides a demonstration of unsupervised learning whereas the latter learns in the presence of a teacher. Most of the literature referencing the BP model stresses that the level of hidden units, F_2, is responsible for learning an associative map between the input level F_1 and the output level F_3. It is the sufficiently distributed nature of this map that allows it to accommodate changes in the input layer and appropriately alter the output layer. Grossberg's (1987a) criticism of the BP model is that the manner in which it carries out its learning renders it inappropriate as a model of the brain. The argument is that self-organization of an associative map can be achieved essentially by a three-level network. Figure 5.6 is essentially a schematic for the ART model architecture. Here the first two levels regulate learning between their bottom-up and top-down pathways and in doing so discover codes with invariant properties in the set of input patterns presented at the lowest level. Activation of these codes at F_2 causes the learning of output patterns at F_3.

In contrast the schematic for the back-propagation model architecture (Fig. 5.7) indicates its relatively greater complexity. The learning proceeds roughly as follows. Inputs at F_1 go through F_2 and generate outputs at F_3. Simultaneously, the expected output is being fed (by an external teacher) to F_4, where the difference between the expected output and the actual output, multiplied by the derivative of the actual output, generates an error signal. This error signal is used to change the weights in the F_2-F_3 pathways. These weights are then communicated to the top-down F_4-F_5 pathways where they are multiplied by the F_4 error signals to generate weighted error signals at F_5. These, appropriately weighted by derivatives as in the layers above, are then used to alter the weights in

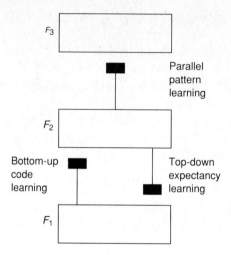

Figure 5.6 *ART model architecture.*

From Grossberg, S. (1987). "Competitive Learning: From Interactive Activation to Adaptive Resonance," Cognitive Science, 11, 23–63. Reprinted with permission of Ablex Publishing Corporation.

the F_1-F_2 pathways. Note that the requirement that outputs be converted to derivatives of outputs at each layer (hence layers F_6 and F_7) adds to the complexity of the entire scheme. Further, note that this entire process is replicated at every stage of BP model hidden units.

Some critical points of difference between the ART and BP models are

1. *Stability of the Learned Code:* Unlike the self-stabilizing nature of the learned code in the ART model, that of the BP model keeps tracking whatever expected outputs are imposed by the teacher and can therefore be unstable in the face of a complex environment.

2. *Expectations as Prototypes:* The absence of a self-scaling property in the BP model prevents it from being able to alter the importance of each expected component when it is embedded in expected outputs of variable complexity. Therefore, instead of gradually discovering invariant characteristic properties of all the exemplars presented to it by the teacher and thus generating a prototype, each exemplar is treated as a prototype. In contrast, the ART model can discover critical feature patterns.

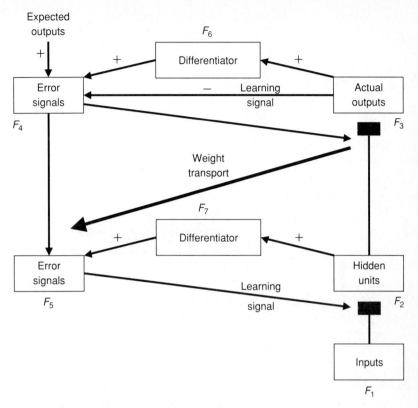

Figure 5.7 *Back-propagation model architecture.*

From Grossberg, S. (1987). "Competitive Learning: From Interactive Activation to Adaptive Resonance," Cognitive Science, 11, 23–63. Reprinted with permission of Ablex Publishing Corporation.

3. *Weight Transport:* As described above, the top-down LTM traces (weights) in the BP model are formal transports of the learned bottom-up LTM traces. This is in contrast to the ART model where the top-down weights are learned by a real-time associative process and are not transports of the bottom-up weights.

4. *Matching to Regulate Learning:* The two-thirds rule in the ART model permits the subliminal sensitizing of the network in preparation for an exemplar of an expected class of input patterns. This helps to regulate learning needed to generate a self-consistent recognition code. In the BP model, however, matching

changes only the weights without having any effect on the fast information-processing accompanying each input trial.

■ 5.9 Literature Overview

The process whereby a simple competitive mechanism is used to extract salient features in a set of input patterns is described in Rumelhart (1985). The material in Section 5.2 is derived from this source, which also provides a brief historical discussion on the factors that stimulated the development of the competitive learning mechanism. A series of experimental results provide useful illustrations of this paradigm's applications.

Linsker (1988) adopts the approach that it should be possible to infer the organizing principles that govern the human perceptual process without necessarily waiting for voluminous quantities of experimental detail that has yet to be uncovered. He cites as an example the fact that it is possible to comprehend the principles of a computer without understanding the functionality of every component. With this in mind, his paper examines the evolution of the property of self-organization in a multilayered network in which the cells operate on the basis of a variation of the Hebbian rule. The material in Section 5.3 is drawn from this source. More details of the mathematics can be obtained from Linsker (1986).

Fukushima (1975), Fukushima (1980), and Fukushima (1986) provide greater mathematical detail and some experimental results related to the cognitron and the neocognitron. These papers are the source of the material in Section 5.4. Similarly, Section 5.5 provides only an introduction to the interaction activation paradigm. The basics of the model proposed by McClelland and Rumelhart are described in McClelland (1981). This article is the source of the material in Section 5.5 and may be consulted for details of experiments that have been used to verify the paradigm. Further extensions to the interactive activation model may be found in a sequel to that paper, Rumelhart (1982).

Grossberg (1987a) offers a comparative analysis of the paradigms that we have considered in this chapter (and a comparison with learning-by-back-propagation that we discussed in Chapter 4). This paper also provides a description of the adaptive resonance paradigm that is proposed as a stabilizing alternative to competitive learning. A more detailed discussion of ART can be found in Carpenter (1988). These papers were the source of the discussion in Sections 5.7 and 5.8.

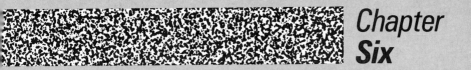

Chapter
Six

The Hopfield and Hoppensteadt Models

■ *6.1 Introduction*

This chapter discusses two broad approaches toward large networks. As Hoppensteadt (1986) mentions, the first of these, the Hopfield net, is based on determining whether a neuron is firing or not, while the second relies primarily on the synchronization of firing frequencies. The discussion of the Hopfield net in the first half of this chapter makes it clear that it can be used not only as an associative memory but also as a solver of optimization problems. The review of the new conceptual framework for computation developed by Hopfield and Tank will complement the development of the theory of associative memory and the distributed representation of information in Chapter 2. While much of the material already covered is not essential to understanding the bare-bones mechanisms that the application architectures introduced below comprise, it is helpful to read the section on Hopfield nets with the theory of associative memory as background. We discuss two applications of Hopfield nets (to the solution of the traveling salesman problem and to problems in vision) in some detail. In view of the resurgence of interest in optical computing, we also provide an introduction to the work being done in developing an optical implementation of the Hopfield net. Finally, there is an important distinction to be made between computational and programming complexity, which is discussed in the context of the Hopfield net solution to the traveling salesman problem.

The second half of the chapter discusses Hoppensteadt's work on controlling large networks by synchronizing firing frequencies. The energy surface approach toward a network of on-off neurons pioneered by the Hopfield net finds an application in Hoppensteadt's networks also. Specifically, Hoppensteadt (1986) shows that it is possible to associate an energy function with phase-locking of a network of electrical oscillators. We provide a brief explanation of phase locking and show how it applies to Hoppensteadt's (1986) network of *voltage controlled oscillator neurons* (VCONs).

Hopfield networks use relaxation techniques to perform multiple-constraint satisfying searches. We make some general comments on relaxation searches and then discuss the application of simulated annealing to Hopfield nets as a way of avoiding getting stuck in a local minimum. Finally, this leads to a brief discussion of the Boltzmann machine learning algorithm.

■ *6.2 The Hopfield-Tank Model*

6.2.1 Biological Background

Hopfield (1986) presents circuits consisting of nonlinear graded-response model neurons organized into networks with effectively symmetric synaptic connections. These circuits, implementable with electronic components, allow complex problems similar to those occurring in biology to be solved without the need to follow the details of the circuit dynamics. Basically, a collection of amplifiers (the details of the most basic circuit are described later) simulates a dense mass of neurons. Resistances and capacitances are used to model "interneuronal" connections. The main thrust of the research here, as has been in the discussion of the various paradigms discussed in Chapters 4 and 5, is the study of the modification of these interconnections so as to simulate a simple, dynamical system.

In early theoretical studies, biological *McCulloch-Pitts neurons* were modeled as logical decision elements described by a two-valued state variable, which were organized into logical decision networks that could compute simple Boolean functions. In general, the McCulloch-Pitts models do not capture two important aspects of biological neurons and circuits: *analog processing* and *high interconnectivity*.

We make the simplifying assumption that the input currents from all channels to individual units in the network are simply additive; more complex interactions between input currents are ignored. Another simplification is to deal only with fast synaptic events (i.e., when a potential fluctuation occurs in the presynaptic terminal of a chemical synapse, a change in the concentration of neurotransmitter is followed, with a slight delay, by a current in the postsynaptic cell—we assume that this delay is much shorter than the membrane time constant of the neuron). Therefore, a change in potential at the soma of cell j introduces an effectively instantaneous conductance change in a postsynaptic cell i. The amount of the conductance change depends on the nature and strength of the synapse from cell j to cell i. The firing rate of cell i can be described by the function $f_i(u_i)$. In the limiting case of a model that suppresses the details of action potentials, two variables describe the state of neuron i: the effective input potential u_i and the output firing rate $f_i(u_i)$. The strength of the synaptic current into a postsynaptic neuron j due to a presynaptic neuron i is proportional to the product of the presynaptic cell's output $[f_i(u_i)]$ and the strength of the synapse from i to j, T_{ij}. This is clearly reminiscent of the Hebbian rule.

6.2.2 Electronic Implementation

Hopfield (1985) provides some details of the electronic circuit that is used to implement this network. Inherent to the system are three sources of parallelism: (1) parallel input channels; (2) parallel output channels; and (3) dense interneuronal, or interamplifier, connectivity.

   The amplifiers that are used to model neurons are characterized by sigmoid, monotonic input-output relations, $V_j = g_j(u_j)$, where V_j and u_j are the output and the input voltages, respectively. The neuronal time-constant is modeled not by the time-constant of the amplifier (which is assumed negligible) but by specific input resistance ρ_j (leading to a reference ground) and an input capacitance c_j. An interneuronal synapse is defined by a conductance T_{ij} (which is implemented by a resistance of value $1/|T_{ij}|$), which connects one of the two outputs of amplifier j (each amplifier is provided with $a+$ and $a-$ output; an excitatory synapse requires the output to be taken from the plus terminal and, an inhibitory synapse requires the output to be taken from the minus terminal) to the input of amplifier i. To model the fact that each neuron computes a nonlinear function of a host of inputs (in the most complete case, the inputs come from the outputs of all the other neurons in the system) under the influence of its own activation level, the electronic model provides a biasing current I_i for each neuron. Essentially these set the general level of excitability of the network (Fig. 6.1).

   The following set of coupled nonlinear differential equations describes the dynamics of an interacting system of N neurons by showing how the neuronal state variables change with time under synaptic current influences.

$$C_i \frac{du_i}{dt} = \sum_{j=1}^{N} T_{ij} V_j - \frac{u_i}{R_i} + I_i,$$

where

$$V_j = g_j(u_j).$$

Here, the R_i is a parallel combination of the input resistance and the resistance used to model synaptic connectivity:

$$\frac{1}{R_i} = \frac{1}{\rho_i} + \sum_{j=1}^{N} \frac{1}{R_{ij}}.$$

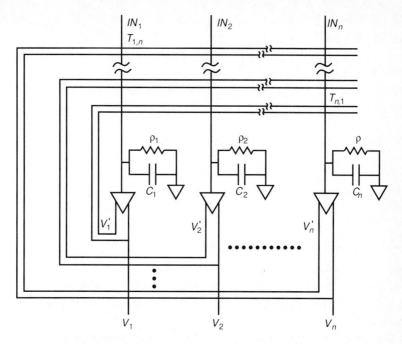

Figure 6.1 *The model neural circuit in electronic components.*

Any neuron's output can potentially be the input of any other neuron. The excitatory and inhibitory
nature of the connection is determined accordingly as the connection is from the normal terminal of an
amplifier to the input of another or from the inverting terminal of the amplifier.

From Hopfield, "Computing with Neural Circuits: A Model," Science, Vol. 233, 625–633. © 1986.
Reprinted with permission.

If for simplicity we assume constant values for the R_i and C_i, and if all
the sigmoid functions g_j are identical, then the equations of motion become

$$\frac{du_i}{dt} = -\frac{u_i}{\tau} + \sum_{j=1}^{N} T_{ij} V_j + I_i,$$

where

$$\tau = RC \quad \text{and}$$

$$V_j = g(u_j).$$

Note that we redefine T_{ij}/C and I_i/C as T_{ij} and I_i, respectively, purely for convenience.

Provided the initial values of the neurons (amplifier states) are specified, this system of equations is capable of completely modeling the time-evolution of the collection of amplifiers. Essential biological features retained include the idea of a neuron as transducer of input to output with a smooth sigmoid response up to a maximum level of output, the integrative behavior of the cell membrane, large numbers of excitatory and inhibitory connections, the reentrant or feedback nature of the connections, and the ability to work with both graded-response neurons and those that produce action potentials. Note especially that the model retains the two important aspects of computation: *dynamics* and *nonlinearity.*

6.2.3 *Discrete versus Continuous-Valued Neural Elements*

Hopfield (1984) demonstrates that neurons with graded response have collective computational properties like those of two-state neurons. The properties of the original McCulloch-Pitts neurons are all preserved in the analog model. This may be seen as some sort of motivation for using analog neural systems to deal with combinatorial problems. While analog systems imply that real circuits using operational amplifiers, resistors, and capacitors can be used to construct a content-addressable memory, the original stochastic model still remains, clearly, very efficient for the purposes of simulation on a digital computer.

Consider the network described above utilizing two-state McCulloch-Pitts neurons. The total input to neuron i is given by

$$H_i = \sum_{j \neq i} T_{ij} V_j + I_i .$$

Now, each neuron samples its inputs stochastically (and independently of all the other neurons). This results in an asynchronous mode of operation (the asynchrony is supposed to represent a combination of propagation delays, jitter, and noise in real neural systems). The change of state rule may be represented thus

$$V_i \rightarrow V_i^0 \quad \text{if } \sum_{j \neq i} T_{ij} V_j + I_i < U_i$$

$$\rightarrow V_i^1 \quad \text{if } \sum_{j \neq i} T_{ij} V_j + I_i > U_i,$$

where U_i is the threshold level and V_i^0 and V_i^1 are the two states of the McCulloch-Pitts neuron.

This system functions as an associative/content-addressable memory as long as the system is characterized by a set of stable states such that when the system is initialized to a position near one of these states, the system evolves to that state. It is shown that convergent flow to stable states is guaranteed when the synaptic conductivity matrix T is symmetric with zero diagonal elements. Consider an "energy" function

$$E = -\frac{1}{2} \sum_{i \neq j} \sum T_{ij} V_i V_j - \sum_i I_i V_i + \sum_i U_i V_i .$$

Any change in any V_i leads to the following change in E:

$$\Delta E = -\left[\sum_{j \neq i} T_{ij} V_j + I_i - U_i \right] \Delta V_i .$$

Since ΔV_i has the same sign as the bracketed term, ΔE is always negative. Further, since E is bounded, sufficient iterations will lead to stable states.

To see that the deterministic case has the same properties in continuous-space flow that the stochastic case has in discrete-space flow, consider the energy function

$$E = -\frac{1}{2} \sum_{i,j} \sum T_{ij} V_i V_j + \sum_i \frac{1}{R_i} \int_0^{V_i} g_i^{-1}(V)\, dV + \sum_i I_i V_i .$$

Consider the time-derivative

$$\frac{dE}{dT} = -\sum_i \frac{dV_i}{dt} \left(\sum_j T_{ij} V_j - \frac{u_i}{R_i} + I_i \right)$$

$$= -\sum_i C_i \frac{dV_i}{dt} \frac{du_i}{dt}$$

$$= -\sum_i C_i g_i^{-1\prime}(V_i) \left(\frac{dV_i}{dt} \right)^2 .$$

Here, C_i is positive and $g_i^{-1}(V_i)$ is monotonic and increasing. Therefore $dE/dt \leq 0$. $dE/dt = 1$ implies that $dV_i/dt = 0$ for all i. Therefore the motion seeks out the minima of E and comes to a stop at such points.

There is a close correspondence between the stable states of the stochastic and the deterministic models. Assume the following for the continuous case. Let $V_i^0 < 0 < V_i^1$; then the zero of voltage for each V_i is chosen so that $g_i(0) = 0$ for all i. Assume asymptotes are at $+1$ and -1 for all i. Let us consider the two terms in the continuous-case energy function separately.

Since E is a linear function of a single V_i along any cube edge, the energy extrema of

$$E = -\frac{1}{2} \sum_{i \neq j} \sum T_{ij} V_i V_j$$

for the discrete space $V_i = +1, -1$ are the same corners as the energy extrema for the continuous case $V_i^0 < 0 < V_i^1$.

In order to study the effect of the steepness of the sigmoid input-output relation on the correspondence of the stable states of the two models, rescale as follows:

$$V_i = g_i(u_i) \qquad \text{by} \qquad V_i = g_i(\lambda u_i)$$

and

$$u_i = g_i^{-1}(V_i) \qquad \text{by} \qquad u_i = \frac{1}{\lambda} g_i^{-1}(V_i).$$

The second term in E (continuous-case) is now given by

$$\frac{1}{\lambda} \sum_i \frac{1}{R_i} \int_0^{V_i} g_i^{-1}(V) \, dV.$$

As V_i approaches $+1, -1$, the integral becomes very large. However, in the very high gain case (λ very large), the entire contribution of this term is negligible. Therefore, the extrema are those caused by only the first term. The only stable points of the very high gain, continuous, deterministic system therefore correspond to the stable points of the stochastic system. When λ does not approach infinity, but is still large, the second term causes the energy surface to have its maxima at the corners and minima slightly displaced toward the interior of the hypercube. As λ becomes smaller, the minima move further inward (there is still one minimum to correspond to each maximum). For further decrease in λ, the minima begin to disappear as they coalesce with a saddle point until for $\lambda = 0$, there is only one minimum at $V_i = 0$.

6.2.4 The Minimal Energy Concept: The Motivation behind Network Dynamics

A general form circuit is described by the value of the synapses T_{ij} and input currents I_i. The state of the system of neurons is defined by the value of the outputs V_i (i.e., output of the amplifier used to model a neuron). In a geometric space with a cartesian axis for each neural output, the instantaneous state is represented by a point. For a circuit with arbitrary values for the synaptic connections, the trajectories of this point can be very complex. A symmetric circuit is defined as having synaptic strength and sign (excitation or inhibition) of the connection from neuron i to j the same as from j to i. Symmetry of the connections results in a powerful theorem (about the system behavior) that shows that a mathematical quantity E, which is interpreted as computational energy, decreases during the change in neural state with time, described by the above equation. This energy is a global quantity not felt by an individual neuron. It is our way of understanding why the system behaves as it does and it is similar to the concept of entropy in a simple gas.

Since, in general, E is minimized as the circuit computes, the dynamics produce a path through the space that tends to minimize the energy and therefore the cost function. Eventually, a stable-state configuration is reached that corresponds to a local minimum of the E function. The solution to the problem is then decoded from this configuration. In the high-gain case (i.e., the sigmoid input-output relation is steep), the energy function is

$$E = -\frac{1}{2} \sum_{i,j} T_{i,j} V_i V_j - \sum_j I_j V_j.$$

6.2.5 Application of Hopfield Nets—The Traveling Salesman Problem

Hopfield (1985, 1986) uses the neural network and its associated energy minimization principle described above to devise a solution to the NP-complete traveling salesman problem. The problem is described as follows. A set of n cities A, B, C, have pairwise distances of separation d_{AB}, $d_{AC}, \ldots, d_{BC}, \ldots$. The aim is to find the shortest closed tour that visits each city once and returns to the starting city. The problem is mapped onto a neural net as follows.

A row vector of length n is used to show the position of a particular city during a tour. Thus if city x is the third city on the tour, then the third entry of the vector is 1 and all the others are 0. Clearly, one such row vector is required for each of the n cities. Put together, we have an n by n matrix. Therefore, the mapped n-city traveling salesman problem requires n^2 neurons. Note further that any permutation matrix represents a tour of the cities (the only requirement for a tour, in terms of matrix entries, is that each row and each column should contain one and only one 1 entry; all other entries should be 0).

Each of the $n!$ permutation matrices corresponds to a valid tour; of these some are of equal length. It turns out that there are $n!/2n$ *distinct paths* for closed traveling salesman problem (TSP) routes. In the derivations that follow, we use symbols of the form $V_{X,j}$ where X is the city name and j is the position of the city in the tour.

The following considerations are important in devising the energy function that is minimized during the computation. States representing permutation matrices should be stable. Further, those $n!/2n$ states that correspond to the shortest tours must be favored states. The energy function is minimized over the 2^N corners of the N-dimensional hypercube defined by each $V_i = 0$ or 1. If the function takes the form

$$
E = \frac{A}{2} \sum_X \sum_i \sum_{j \neq i} V_{X,i} V_{X,j} + \frac{B}{2} \sum_i \sum_X \sum_{X \neq Y} V_{X,i} V_{X,j}
$$

$$
+ \frac{C}{2} \left(\sum_X \sum_i V_{X,i} - n \right)^2 + \frac{1}{2} D \sum_X \sum_{X \neq Y} \sum_i d_{X,Y} V_{X,i} (V_{Y,i+1} + V_{Y,i-1}),
$$

where

$A, B, C > 0 ;$

then, each of the four terms in the expression for E above have a direct physical interpretation.

1. Term 1 is 0 if and only if each city row contains no more than one 1.

2. Term 2 is 0 if and only if each tour-position column contains no more than one 1.

Note that the above two conditions define a permutation matrix.

3. Term 3 is 0 if and only if there are n entries of 1 in the entire matrix.

4. Term 4 is minimized when the length of the tour is minimized.

Combining the above, we see that if A, B, and C are sufficiently large, the low-energy states of a network will form a valid tour. The total energy of a valid state will be the length of the tour, and the states with the shortest path will be the lowest-energy states.

The synaptic connectivities can now be expressed in terms of the energy function terms as follows:

$$T_{Xi,Yj} = -A\delta_{XY}(1 - \delta_{ij})$$ inhibitory connections within a row

$$= -B\delta_{ij}(1 - \delta_{XY})$$ inhibitory connections within a column

$$= -C$$ global inhibition

$$= -Dd_{XY}(\delta_{j,i+1} + \delta_{j,i-1})$$ data term,

where

$$\delta_{ij} = 1 \quad \text{if } i = j \quad \text{and} \quad 0 \text{ otherwise.}$$

Finally, the input biasing currents are given by

$$I_{X,i} = Cn.$$

It is insightful to consider the benefits of moving away from the discrete McCulloch-Pitts neurons to the continuous sigmoid input-output function. An observation of the state of the n^2 neurons at an arbitrary time need not yield a permutation matrix. As is explained by Hopfield (1985), the actual domain of the network function is the entire hypercube (i.e., including the interior and not just the vertices). Whenever the function is not at one of the vertices, there is at least one neuron whose output value is neither 0 nor 1 but lies somewhere in-between. Such "nebulous-state" neurons indicate the *likelihood* of a particular city being in a particular position in the tour. Thus if neurons $(2, 3)$ and $(2, 6)$ have outputs between 0 and 1, then the system is simultaneously considering the possibility of the second city being visited in either of position 3 or 6. *It is precisely this simultaneous consideration of several tours that makes the system efficient.* The decision making process consists therefore of a smooth motion from an initial point in the interior of the n-dimensional hypercube to a point sufficiently close to a vertex of the hypercube to be identifiable with that vertex. At any interior point (where the notion of a tour is really undefined), at least one city could be in more than one position in the tour with different likelihoods. A more complete discussion of the use of graded response neurons versus binary state neurons has been provided in Section 6.2.4.

This is a good time to make mention of some recent work by Platt (1987) in the field of constrained differential optimization. External criteria sometimes restrict the acceptable output space in optimization problems. Thus, the unconstrained version of the traveling salesman problem would require that the total travel distance be minimized. The constraint that is imposed in the version that we are considering is that the salesman visit each city exactly once. In general, a constrained optimization problem can be expressed as follows: minimize $f(\bar{x})$ and subject to $g(\bar{x}) = 0$, where $\bar{x}$ denotes the state of the neural network. The evolution of the state during constrained optimization should be such that it should be attracted to the constraining subspace and should then slide along until it finds the locally smallest occurrence of the function f.

Conventional approaches to dealing with constrained optimization include the penalty method and the Lagrange multiplier method. Both of these convert the constrained problem into an unconstrained one. In the former, the unconstrained version is

$$\text{minimize } \varepsilon_{\text{penalty}}(\bar{x}) = f(\bar{x}) + c(g(\bar{x}))^2.$$

As c becomes very large, this method is globally convergent to the required minimum of function f. In the Lagrange multiplier method, consider

$$\varepsilon_{\text{lagrange}}(\bar{x}) = f(\bar{x}) + \lambda g(\bar{x}).$$

Now, a solution to the original function is a critical point of $\varepsilon_{\text{lagrange}}$.

The method proposed by Platt (1987), the *basic differential multiplier method* (BDMM), is a creative alternative to the differential gradient descent that estimates Lagrange multipliers. Gradient descent techniques applied to $\varepsilon_{\text{lagrange}}$ yield

$$x_i' = -\frac{\delta \varepsilon_{\text{lagrange}}}{\delta x_i} = -\frac{\delta f}{\delta x_i} - \lambda \frac{\delta g}{\delta x_i}$$

$$\lambda' = -\frac{\delta \varepsilon_{\text{lagrange}}}{\delta \lambda} = -g(\bar{x}).$$

Unfortunately, since a critical point of $\varepsilon_{\text{lagrange}}$ need not be an attractor for this system, gradient descent techniques do not work with Lagrange multipliers. However, a simple change that allows gradient ascent on λ ensures that the critical points of $\varepsilon_{\text{lagrange}}$ are attractors for the following differential equations (which also solve the initial constrained optimization problem):

$$x_i' = -\frac{\delta f}{\delta x_i} - \lambda \frac{\delta g}{\delta x_i}$$

$$\lambda' = +g(\bar{x}).$$

These equations constitute the BDMM. To see that this system is, in fact, one that undergoes damped oscillations, combine the differential equations to get

$$x_i'' + \sum_j \left(\frac{\delta^2 f}{\delta x_i \, \delta x_j} + \lambda \frac{\delta^2 g}{\delta x_i \, \delta x_j} \right) x_j' + g \frac{\delta g}{\delta x_i} = 0.$$

The damping matrix in this system is given by

$$A_{ij} = \frac{\delta^2 f}{\delta x_i \, \delta x_j} + \lambda \frac{\delta^2 g}{\delta x_i \, \delta x_j}.$$

Without going into details, it is sufficient to say that it can be shown that BDMM always converges whenever the constrained optimization problem has a quadratic function f and the constraint function g is a piecewise linear continuous function. Such a case has given the name quadratic programming.

BDMM has been used to find a good solution to the planar traveling salesman problem. The elements of a discretized "snake" curve are points on the plane, (x_i, y_i). The object is to

$$\text{minimize } \sum_i (x_{i+1} - x_i)^2 - (y_{i+1} - y_i)^2$$

subject to

$$k(x^* - x_c) = 0 \quad \text{and} \quad k(y^* - y_c) = 0.$$

Here (x^*, y^*) are city coordinates and (x_c, y_c) are snake points closest to the city. The important thing to note is this is a quadratic program and BDMM is therefore a useful technique to apply.

The traveling salesman problem provides an excellent opportunity for illustrating the use of neural-net techniques to solve difficult optimization problems. In the particular case of this problem, it is worth recalling that there do exist excellent heuristics that outperform neural-net techniques. Consider as an example the case where the cities obey the triangle inequality (i.e., the direct distance between any two cities is less than that between the same two cities through a third city). View the problem instance as a graph with the cities as vertices and the edges labeled with the intercity distances. There exist polynomial time algorithms to find the minimum spanning tree of such a graph (in the jargon of graph theory, a spanning tree of a graph is a subgraph with all the vertices of the original graph and enough of the edges such that all the vertices are connected and such that there exists exactly one path between any pair of vertices). The suggested heuristic for converting a minimum spanning tree into a good solution for the traveling salesman problem involves visiting all the cities by traversing twice around the tree and using some clever shortcuts permitted by the triangle inequality to get a tour that is no longer than twice that provided by an optimal solution to the traveling salesman problem. This heuristic has been improved by Christofides's use of matching techniques and Eulerian tours so that the heuristic yields a tour that is no longer than 1.5 times that provided by the optimal solution. Garey (1979) may be consulted for details of these and other heuristics.

6.2.6 Application of Hopfield Nets—Problems in Vision

Koch (1986) explores the applications of Hopfield nets to problems in vision. Depth computation from stereoscopic vision, reconstructing and smoothing images from sparse data, and motion computation are vision problems that can be solved using *standard regularization theory*. This technique solves these problems in terms of quadratic energy functionals that must be minimized. One example of a problem well suited to this method is that of smooth surface reconstruction. Typically, the depth values of the object are given only at certain points (alternatively, enough depth values may be available but the data might be very noisy). Basically, the object's surface has to be interpolated between the points where data is not available. This corresponds to finding a best-fit surface between the points. The energy or cost function to be minimized $E(f)$, derived from the inverse problem,

$$Bf = d + n$$

where

d = data,
n = noise, and
B = linear operator

is given by

$$E(f) = \|Bf - d\|^2 + \alpha\|Sf\|^2$$

B and d are known, f is to be computed. The first term in $E(f)$ indicates the distance from the solution to the data and the second term corresponds to a regularizer needed to make the problem well posed. For surface interpolation, B is a diagonal matrix with elements equal to 1 at those locations where depth is known and 0 otherwise. Koch (1986) shows that E can be redefined as

$$L(V) = \frac{1}{2} \sum_{i,j} T_{ij} V_i V_j + \sum_i V_i I_i .$$

This redefinition requires replacing

T by $2(B^T B + \alpha S^T S)$,
V by f,
I_i by $-2B^T d$,

and dropping the constant term $d^T d$. (The symbols have the same meaning that they had in the development of the traveling salesman neural net solution). Every neuron is grounded with a resistance, and a capacitance is put in parallel with it. The expression for L can be interpreted as the Lyapunov function of the network. Change in the potential is given by

$$C_i \frac{dV_i}{dt} = -\frac{\partial L}{\partial V_i}.$$

Quadratic variational principles that can be expressed in the form that $E(f)$ is expressed above and can be solved with an appropriate electrical network, where the connections can be implemented by linear ohmic resistances and the data by injected currents.

Standard regularization theory can be applied only to convex energy functions. Consequently, the technique described above cannot be used to deal with discontinuities (e.g., the surface interpolation scheme used in smooth surface reconstruction would not function when discontinuities are present). Koch (1986) presents an extension to the Hopfield technique in the form of *line processes*. The idea behind this process is as follows. For surface reconstruction, for example, two coupled Markov random fields are used to model the surface. One is a continuous-valued field that corresponds to the depth f_i at location i. The other is a binary field (line process) whose variables, located at sites between the depth lattice, indicate whether a discontinuity is present between two depth lattice points or not. Bayesian theory shows that the best estimate of the surface corresponds to the global minimization of an energy function that, in one dimension, is given by

$$E(f, h) = \sum_i (f_{i+1} - f_i)^2 (1 - h_i) + c_D \sum_i (f_i - d_i)^2 + c_L \sum_i h_i,$$

where h_i is the binary line process.

The h_i introduce local minima into the energy function and make it nonquadratic. Following Hopfield (1984), Koch (1986) maps the binary line processes into continuous variables bounded by 0 and 1. The resulting energy function is shown to be minimized at the corners of the hypercube (even though the energy function contains cubic terms).

6.2.7 Reduction of Oscillatory Phenomena in Hopfield Nets[1]

We have described above Hopfield and Tank's electronic implementation of a neural network. It is interesting to see how researchers have dealt with the practical issues that come up in the actual implementation of the model. For instance, real problems deal with numbers and therefore there must be a way of specifying numbers in a neural network. There is a brief discussion of this issue in the next section. As another example, Takeda (1986) points out that, in the discrete time model that they used, oscillatory behavior arises when T_{ii} is different from zero. This can hamper convergence to the minima in the state space. They adopted four discrete-time transition modes in an attempt to reduce this oscillation. These are described below (see Fig. 6.2).

[1]From Takeda, "Neural Networks for Computation: Number Representations and Programming Complexity," *Applied Optics*, Vol. 25, No. 18, 134–136, September 1986. Reprinted with permission from the American Institute of Physics.

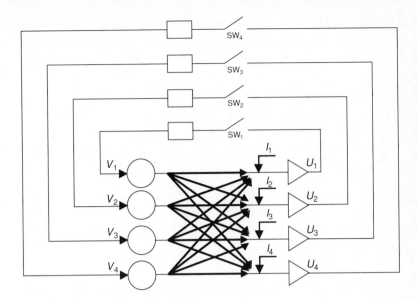

Figure 6.2 *A neural network model.*

V_i and U_i are the input and output potentials respectively. I_i are the biasing currents. The pattern with which the switches SW_i are closed determines the transition mode being used in the model.

From Takeda, "Neural Networks for Computation: Number Representations and Programming Complexity," Applied Optics, 25, No. 18, 3033–3046. © 1986 American Institute of Physics. Reprinted with permission.

Direct Synchronous Transition Mode. Switches SW_i turn on in synchrony to cause simultaneous transitions at discrete times k. A continuous nonlinear function $g(x)$ allows neurons to assume values between 0 and 1.

$$U_i(k) = \sum_{j=1}^{N} T_{ij} V_j(k) + I_i$$

$$V_i(k + 1) = g[U_i(k)].$$

Differential Synchronous Transition Mode. Transitions occur synchronously but this time are governed by difference equations. The hardware implication for this method is that each neuron needs a memory cell to keep its previous input.

$$U_i(k) - U_i(k - 1) = \sum_{j=1}^{N} T_{ij} V_j(k) + I_i$$

$$V_i(k + 1) = g[U_i(k)].$$

Direct Asynchronous Transition Mode (Random Delays). The only difference between this mode and the direct synchronous transition mode is that the switches turn on and off asynchronously (i.e., with random delays).

$$U_i(k - \Delta t_i) = \sum_{j=1}^{N} T_{ij} V_j(k - \Delta t_i) + I_i$$

$$V_i(k - \Delta t_i + \varepsilon) = g[U_i(k - \Delta t_i)],$$

where

Δt_i = time-delay induced skews (fraction of a clock cycle) and

ε = small positive constant.

Here, there is no need for a particular neuron to wait for all the others to be updated before it updates itself. It can also make use of information about new states of other neurons that have already renewed their states.

Differential Asynchronous Transition Mode (Random Delays). This is the asynchronous version of the differential synchronous transition mode.

$$U_i(k - \Delta t_i) - U_i(k - \Delta t_i - 1) = \sum_{j=1}^{N} T_{ij} V_j(k - \Delta t_i) + I_i$$

$$V_i(k - \Delta t_i + \varepsilon) = g[U_i(k - \Delta t_i) - U_i(k - \Delta t_i - 1)].$$

In the case where T_{ii} is different from zero the synchronous methods did not provide a solution to the oscillatory problem. Therefore, a proper choice should depend on the application and should ideally be made from either the direct or the differential asynchronous transition mode.

6.2.8 Representation of Numbers in Neural Space[2]

Takeda (1986) has suggested three different ways of mapping the positive integer space Z^+ onto the neuron state space V. In all three schemes, linear combinations of neuron-state variables are used to represent numbers.

[2]From Takeda, "Neural Networks for Computation: Number Representations and Programming Complexity," *Applied Optics*, 25, No. 18, September 1986. Reprinted with permission of the American Institute of Physics.

Note that the Hopfield energy function is quadratic with respect to the neuron-state variables. Nonlinear mappings from the number space onto the neuron-state space cannot form the Hopfield energy function because the floating point expressions have neuron state variables as exponents.

Binary Scheme. The binary scheme uses binary digits to represent a number. This method requires $\log_2(N + 1)$ bits to express a number N. There is a one-to-one correspondence between the numbers and their representations. Since not only a particular neuronal state but also the neuronal position (i.e., units digit, tens digit, etc.) are critical in determining the correct numeral, this representation is particularly susceptible to faults.

Simple Sum Scheme. In the simple sum scheme a number N is represented by the sum of the neuron-state variables. Therefore 3 can be represented by 11001, 00111, 10101, and so on. Clearly this is a one-to-many mapping. Also, N neurons are required to represent a number N. Since there are many mappings for each number, the system is highly fault-tolerant. This system also has a greater problem solving capability. In contrast to the binary scheme, where only one point in the state space gives the correct solution, here multiple points provide correct answers. This suggests a greater likelihood of getting the answer.

Group-and-Weight Scheme. To benefit from the superior capability of the simple sum scheme and to avoid some of the problem of requiring too many neurons for large numbers, a compromise between the two schemes mentioned above is suggested — the group-and-weight scheme. The total q bits are divided into K groups each with M bits (i.e., $q = KM$). The groups are interpreted as digits whose numbers are given by simple sums of the bits in the corresponding groups. Therefore an expression for the value of the q bits is given by

$$\sum_{k=1}^{K} \left[(M + 1)^{k-1} \sum_{i=1}^{M} V_{(k-1)M+i} \right].$$

$M = 1, K = q$ reduces the expression to the binary form,

$$\sum_{k=1}^{q} 2^{k-1} V_k.$$

$M = q$, $K = 1$ reduces the expression to the simple-sum form,

$$\sum_{i=1}^{q} V_i.$$

The group-and-weight scheme requires $\log_{M+1}(N + 1)$ bits to express a number N.

The group-and-weight scheme can be used to represent bipolar and complex integers too. Bipolar numbers are obtained by adding a negative bias integer to the positive integer expression. Thus,

$$\sum_{k=1}^{K} \left[(M + 1)^{k-1} \sum_{i=1}^{M} V_{(k-1)M+i} \right] - \text{ceiling} \left\{ \frac{1}{2} [(M + 1)^K - 1] \right\},$$

where the second term is half of the largest positive integer that can be expressed by the first term and ceiling (x) gives the smallest integer $\geq x$.

Note that the range over which numbers can be expressed is now given by

$$\pm \frac{1}{2} [(M + 1)^K - 1].$$

To express complex integers, we need twice as many neurons to express the real and the imaginary parts separately.

Finally, we can represent fractions by using more neurons and labeling them with negative subscripts ($i < 0$) so that the number representation now becomes

$$\sum_{k=-K'}^{K} \left[(M + 1)^{k-1} \sum_{i=1}^{M} V_{(k-1)M+i} \right].$$

Numbers ranging from 0 to $(M + 1)^K - (M + 1)^{-(K'+1)}$ with a minimum digit quantization of $(M + 1)^{-(K'+1)}$ can now be expressed.

6.2.9 *Computational and Programming Complexity*

There is a crucial distinction to be made between computational and programming complexity. Much optimism has arisen from the fact that the convergence time of a neural network is very low, usually of the order of a few iterations. At the present time, insufficient knowledge is available regarding the relationships between convergence time, problem size (reflected in the number of neurons employed in the network), and the algorithm used (pattern of interconnections used). The concepts of associative memory and distributed representation of information have all too important a role to play in the argument that computation time does not grow rapidly with problem size because a larger number of neurons (hence, a higher degree of parallelism) participate in the solution to a larger problem. However, this does not take into consideration the programming time (i.e., the time required to actually implement the algorithm in hardware). This issue is discussed in some detail in Takeda (1986).

Programming complexity is defined as the number of arithmetic operations that must be performed to determine the proper interconnection strengths and neural biases for the problem to be solved. Unlike classical von Neumann machines (with separate memory and processor structures), where a program once implemented and stored in memory can be used to act upon several sets of data, in neural-network computers the program and data are stored in a nondistinguishable fashion in the interconnection strengths and neuronal input biases. These must be altered for each problem instance. Clearly, programming complexity is more important for neural computation. On the other hand, computational complexity (roughly speaking, the number of steps that the algorithm requires to obtain an answer) is the more appropriate measure for von Neumann machines. Studying the relative programming and computational complexities of two examples serves to justify Takeda's (1986) cautionary statement that different problems may or may not require neural networks for their efficient resolution.

As a first example, the traveling salesman problem is examined. Takeda (1986) argues that the problem's computational complexity is $O(N!)$, where N is the number of cities. The Hopfield and Tank solution requires only N^2 neurons to be programmed in $O(N^3)$ time. Here, the vastly greater computational complexity makes it worthwhile to invest in a neural-network implementation. Here we must add our own qualifying remarks. First, the neural-net implementation does not guarantee the best solution. An approximate solution can be obtained in far less than $O(N!)$ time by various clever (non–neural-net) heuristics. Therefore, more precise problem requirements would have to be taken into consideration in deciding whether a neural-net implementation is worthwhile or not.

As another example, consider the solution of N simultaneous equations in N unknowns. In a neural-net implementation where q neurons are used to represent each variable, there are a total of qN neurons with $qN(qN + 1)/2 = O(N^2)$ interconnections. Since it takes $O(N)$ time to determine each interconnection strength, therefore programming complexity is $O(N^3)$. But, the algorithm itself is also an $O(N^3)$ algorithm (i.e., computational complexity). Therefore, there appears to be no advantage to using a neural-network computer over a conventional one.

6.2.10 Optical Implementation of Neural Networks[3]

Since optical signals can flow through three-dimensional space, they are in a better position (than VLSI techniques, where all the wires have to be routed on a planar surface) to imitate the dense interconnections that characterize the human brain. This idea has spawned a body of litera-ture in, for instance, optical applications to Hopfield nets. Some of this is discussed below.

Farhat (1985) and Psaltis (1985) have devised an optical implementa-tion of the Hopfield network (see Fig. 6.3). They point out that the *associ-ating action* of associative memory is basically a nearest-neighbor search. Optical components are used to represent binary neurons (note that these components are either on or off; there are no intermediate stages). The theory behind their implementation is very similar to the standard associative memory theories, but it is presented below for completeness. It is worth noting that the construction of optical content-addressable memories could be greatly simplified by the use of optical bistability devices, bistable light amplifiers with internal feedback, and other avail-able technology. This could open up the possibility for more general com-putations than nearest-neighbor searches in future generation computers.

M N-dimensional, bipolar, binary $(1, -1)$ vectors $v_i^{(m)}$ (referred to as the nominal state vectors) are stored as

$$T_{ij} = \sum_{m=1}^{M} v_i^{(m)} v_j^{(m)} \qquad i, j = 1, 2, \ldots, N \qquad T_{ii} = 0.$$

If the memory is addressed by multiplying the matrix T_{ij} by one of the state vectors, say $v_i^{(m0)}$, we have the estimate

$$\hat{v}_i^{(m0)} = \sum_{j=1}^{N} T_{ij} v_j^{(m0)}$$

$$= \sum_{j \neq i}^{N} \sum_{m=1}^{M} v_i^{(m)} v_j^{(m)} v_j^{(m0)}$$

$$= (N - 1) v_i^{(m0)} + \sum_{m \neq m0} \alpha_{m, m0} v_i^{(m)},$$

[3]Math in Section 6.2.10 from Farhat, "Optical Implementation of Hopfield Model," *Applied Optics*, 24, No. 10, May 1985. Reprinted with permission of the American Institute of Physics.

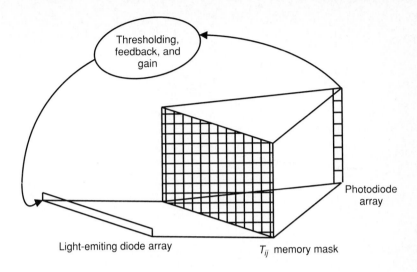

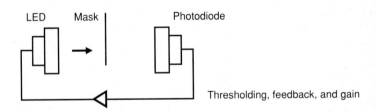

Figure 6.3 *Matrix-vector multiplier incorporating nonlinear electronic feedback.*

From Farhat, "Optical Implementation of the Hopfield Model," Applied Optics, Vol. 24, No. 10, May 1985. Reprinted with permission.

where

$$\alpha_{m,m0} = \sum_{j=1}^{N} v_j^{(m0)} v_j^{(m)}.$$

Here, the second of the output terms represents unwanted cross-talk and, on the average, has a value of $[(M - 1)(N - 1)]^{0.5}$. If N is sufficiently larger than M, then the elements of the estimated vector will be positive if the corresponding elements of $v_i^{(m0)}$ are equal to +1 and negative otherwise. Thresholding of the output vector therefore yields

$$v_i^{(m0)} = \text{sgn}[\hat{v}_i^{(m0)}] = \begin{cases} +1 & \text{if } \hat{v}_i^{(m0)} > 0 \\ -1 & \text{otherwise.} \end{cases}$$

The output vector is an approximation of the stored word that is at the shortest Hamming distance from the input vector. Feeding back the output as a new input results in a new output that generally more accurately represents the stored vector.

The salient features of one of the optical implementations follows. Briefly, an array of light-emitting diodes (LEDs) (each element of the array is capable of representing the component of a unipolar binary vector) represents the neuronal elements. Global interconnections are implemented through the addition of thresholding, gain, and feedback to a conventional optical vector-matrix multiplier. The LED array represents the input vector, the photodiode (PD) array detects the output vector. The output is thresholded and fed back in parallel to drive the corresponding elements of the LED array. Though the implementation above uses electronic feedback, Farhat (1985) points out that it is preferable to use optical feedback by combining the PD and LED arrays into a single compact hybrid [that also contains integrated circuits (ICs) for the nonlinear feedback operation and for the driving of the LEDs]. Arrays of nonlinear, internal-feedback optical light amplifiers or optical bistability devices (OBDs) can replace the PD/LED combination arrays. The resulting content-addressable memory structure is very compact.

It is interesting to note that there has been a resurgence toward developing optical implementations using associative memory. Compare the architecture of a proposed optical computer with that of a conventional one in Figs. 6.4 and 6.5. According to Mada (1985), the change exemplifies the shift from viewing the computer as a model of the brain's calculating ability (conventional computer) to a model of the brain's higher-level information processing ability (optical computer).

■ 6.3 The Hoppensteadt Model[4]

6.3.1 Introduction

Hoppensteadt (1986) adopts the belief that neurons are basic timers in our bodies that also play a central role in storing and processing infor-

[4]Adapted from F.C. Hoppensteadt, *An Introduction to the Mathematics of Neurons*, New York: Cambridge University Press, © 1986. Reprinted with permission of Cambridge University Press.

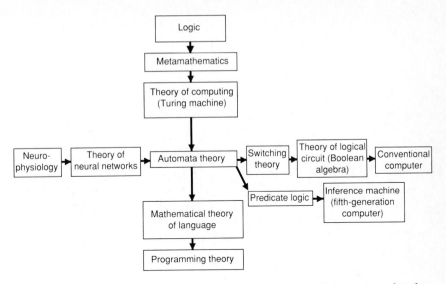

Figure 6.4 *Block diagram of the fundamental principle of the conventional computer.*

From Mada, "Architecture for Optical Computing Using Holographic Associative Memories," Applied Optics, Vol. 24, No. 14, July 1985. Reprinted with permission of the American Institute of Physics.

mation in the brain. The approach of this work is to emphasize the frequency (phase) information of the timers by deriving a model for firing phases of neurons. This electrical model is called a voltage controlled oscillator neuron (VCON), and differs from earlier conventional neuron models in that it is specifically designed to facilitate the study of neuronal frequency-response properties. Some of the earlier models include the Hodgkin-Huxley model, the FitzHugh-Nagumo model, and a simple integrate-and-fire model. All of these employ the method of building up a charge to a certain point and then releasing it within a circuit. In contrast, the VCON network, made possible by integrated circuitry, is modeled by a voltage controlled oscillator feedback loop, representing the neuron body, and a filter in series with a clipping amplifier, representing a chemical synapse. This shall be discussed in some detail later.

Just as Hopfield has derived energy surfaces for his networks of on-off neurons, Hoppensteadt shows that it is possible to associate an energy function with phase-locking of a network of electrical oscillators (i.e., VCONs). Thus, as in the Hopfield networks, short-term memory can be represented by stable firing patterns. While the Hopfield nets incorporated an asynchronous sampling structure and used a convenient measure of energy, they suffered from drawbacks that VCON networks are

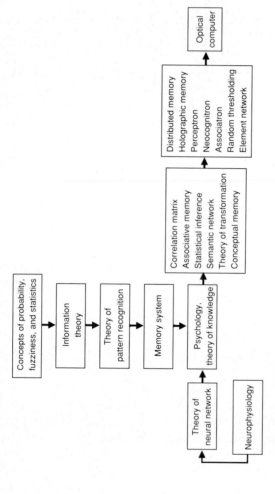

Figure 6.5 Tentative block diagram for the optical computer.

From Mada, "Architecture for Optical Computing Using Holographic Associative Memories," Applied Optics, Vol. 24, No. 14, July 1985. Reprinted with permission of the American Institute of Physics.

able to circumvent to a greater or lesser degree. As an example, Hopfield nets have no spatial structure built into them. Thus, no a priori restrictions are imposed on the connection matrix. Also, since neuron sampling is done statistically, not only does the neuron have to wait for an above-threshold stimulation, but it also has to wait to be sampled. Hopfield's model also suffers from the drawback that it does not lend itself easily to mathematical analysis and, therefore, reliance must be placed on computer simulations.

6.3.2 A Few Words on Neuron Physiology

When a semipermeable membrane separates regions having differing concentrations of an electrically charged chemical species, a potential difference is established across the membrane. The Nernst equation is used to calculate this potential difference:

$$E = \left(\frac{kT}{q}\right) \log\left(\frac{C_1}{C_2}\right),$$

where

> k is a gas constant,
> T is the absolute temperature,
> q is the ionic charge, and
> C_1 and C_2 are the ionic concentrations on the membrane's two sides.

Dendrites receive signals and convey them to the cell body that generates a voltage pulse called an action potential. This pulse is carried by the axon to the synapse (see Fig. 6.6). The latter releases neurotransmitters that diffuse through the synaptic gap to the dendrite of some other neuron, where they create an electric potential across the dendrite's membrane. This potential, if above the neuron's threshold, causes the cell body to fire (i.e., generate an action potential). Sodium (Na^+) and potassium (K^+) ions are the ones most important to cell membrane potential. Neuron membranes at rest are impermeable to sodium. So the observed potential is near E_K. When the membrane is excited, it becomes permeable to sodium, and the channel potential approaches E_{Na} quickly. The potassium diffuses less rapidly but eventually returns the membrane potentials to near E_K again.

Let $c(t)$ denote the concentration of neurotransmitter in the synaptic gap. This increases when action potentials arriving at the synapse

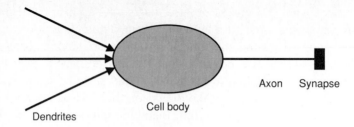

Figure 6.6 *Diagram of neuron physiology.*

stimulate release of neurotransmitter into the gap. Some of the neuro-transmitter binds with the postsynaptic membrane, some diffuses out of the synaptic gap. These chemical kinetics are modeled thus

$$\frac{dc}{dt} = -k_{\mathrm{diff}}c - k_{\mathrm{post}}c + S,$$

where

k_{diff} is the rate constant for diffusion out of the synaptic gap,
k_{post} is the rate constant for combination with postsynaptic membrane, and
S is the source that releases neurotransmitter into the synaptic gap.

6.3.3 VCON: A Voltage-Controlled Oscillator Analog of a Neuron

Hoppensteadt has modeled the cell body as a voltage-controlled oscillator (VCO) (Fig. 6.7). The equation governing the feedback loop is

$$\frac{dx_v}{dt} = e_0 + \omega_0$$

where

x_v is the phase,
e_0 is the acquisition voltage, and
ω_0 is the VCO's center frequency.

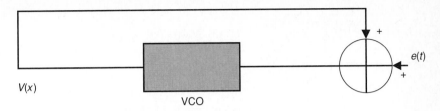

$V(x)$ VCO $e(t)$

Figure 6.7 *VCO modeled as an analog of a neuron.*

Reprinted with the permission of Cambridge University Press.

V is interpreted as the cell body's membrane potential and can be any continuously differentiable function that is 2π periodic in x.

The synapse is modeled by an analog circuit, SYN, as shown in Fig. 6.8 and described below. Action potentials, as described above, range from E_K (approximately -70 mV) to E_{Na} (approximately 55 mV). To incorporate the fact that there is a threshold voltage below which the neuron will not fire, the first device in the SYN analog circuit is a diode. Hoppensteadt assumes that the interaction of the neurotransmitter (released into the synaptic gap) with the postsynaptic membrane is modeled by adding the effect of the neurotransmitter to the existing postsynaptic potential and trimming the sum to fit the membrane's physiological limits. This is done using a comparison amplifier.

The VCON is the combination of the SYN and the VCO as shown in Fig. 6.9.

Figure 6.8 *The synapse modeled by an analog circuit.*

Reprinted with the permission of Cambridge University Press.

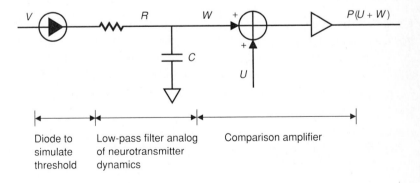

Diode to simulate threshold | Low-pass filter analog of neurotransmitter dynamics | Comparison amplifier

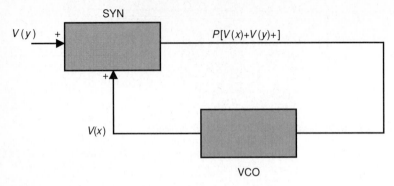

Figure 6.9 *Diagrammatic representation of the VCON.*

Reprinted with the permission of Cambridge University Press.

6.3.4 Clocks and Phase Locking

An analogy can be drawn between biological and mechanical clocks. The latter are primarily comprised of (1) an escapement, a regular beat-setting mechanism; (2) a modulator, a mechanism that translates the escapement's beat into observable motion; and (3) a clock face, a surface where the modulated beat can be observed. Neurons function as the escapements of biological clocks. Muscles and glands scale the time by averaging neuron output. Finally, the effects of such scaling are visible through bodily functions such as respiration.

Consider a simple single-handed clock. We choose the angular distance of its hand from its resting position ϕ as a measure of elapsed time. Then we might say that

$$\frac{d\phi}{dt} = \alpha.$$

Therefore, the rate of change of ϕ is α. While we may think of the simple clock as being driven by a motor that generates the rate α, it is clear (from the manner in which the rate of bodily functions changes under differing circumstances) that the human body perceives time differently. A modulated simple clock is a more appropriate model for the body clock and is described thus,

$$\frac{d\phi}{dt} = \alpha + f\left(\frac{2\pi t}{1440}\right),$$

where f has period 2π. f passes through one complete cycle in the course of the 1440 minutes that comprise a day. In general, we can model a clock whose modulation can come from several sources (outside signals, clock phase feedback, and interaction with other clocks) thus,

$$\frac{d\phi}{dt} = \alpha + F(t, \phi, \psi_1, \psi_2, \ldots, \psi_n),$$

where

$\psi_1, \psi_2, \ldots, \psi_n$ are the phases of other clocks that affect this one.

Hoppensteadt shows that VCON neural networks are governed by equations having the same form.

Neurons are coupled by the chemical activity that occurs between the neurotransmitter that is released into the synaptic gap and the post-synaptic membrane. Since we have been studying the timing aspects of a neuron's functioning, it is instructive to study methods whereby clocks can be coupled. To realize the relevance of studying coupling, note that biological clocks all operate in a common chemical bath and, therefore, must be synchronized. This brings us to the idea of *phase locking,* a phenomenon that explains how large, complicated networks can synchronize in stable ways. To provide an intuitive grasp of this concept, Hoppensteadt uses the example of the notes on a piano being made by using one hammer to strike three wires. Now, though all three wires cannot be tuned in exactly the same fashion, if they are tuned closely enough, then, due to phase locking, they will vibrate at the same frequency when struck. Alternatively, several pendulum clocks mounted on a wall are synchronized by subtle vibrations in the wall and even in the air.

Phase-locked loops (PLL) are, in fact, very basic parts of electronic timing circuits. Studying the rudiments of a PLL shows that a VCON is indeed a PLL. It is essential to introduce some definitions of basic electronic circuits to demonstrate this fact.

A *phase detector circuit* has as its output a periodic function of the phase difference between its two oscillatory inputs. Figure 6.10(a) shows an input signal with phase x_{in} being compared to a reference signal of phase x_{ref}. In the general schematic diagram Fig. 6.10(b), $V(x)$ is a voltage having phase x, V has period 2π, Q is a periodic phase detector characteristic with $Q(0) = 0$, and

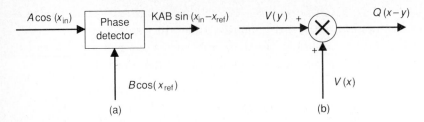

(a) (b)

Figure 6.10 *The phase detector circuit: (a) input signal compared with reference signal; and (b) schematic diagram.*

$$\int_0^{2\pi} Q(x)\, dx = 0\,.$$

A VCO incorporates its controlling voltage in its output phase as shown in Fig. 6.11.

The model for the basic phase-locked loop circuit (Fig. 6.12) is clarified by tracing around the loop.

$$z(t) = \tilde{k}(p)A\,\sin(x_{in} - x_{VCO})$$

$$x_{VCO} = \omega_{VCO}t + \int_0^t (z(s) + e(s))\, ds\,.$$

Note that here $\tilde{k}(p)$ is the Laplace transform of the function $k(t)$ and is given by

$$\tilde{k}(p) = \int_0^\infty e^{-pt} k(t)\, dt\,.$$

Figure 6.11 *VCO with the controlling voltage in the output phase.*

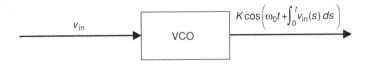

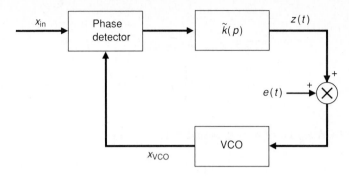

Figure 6.12 *Model for the basic phase-locked loop circuit.*

Reprinted with the permission of Cambridge University Press.

For a constant acquisition voltage $(e(t) = e_0)$, $x_{in} = w^*t$, and no filter present $[(i.e., \tilde{k}(p) = 1)]$, we have

$$\frac{dx_{in}}{dt} = w^*$$

$$\frac{dx_{VCO}}{dt} = e_0 + \omega_0 + A\ \sin(x_{in} - x_{VCO}).$$

A mixer (Fig. 6.13) is a combination of frequency multipliers and dividers and phase detectors. Basically, the two input phases, x and y, and all of their harmonic combinations are compared. Here $n = (n_1, n_2)$ is a multiindex and B_n is the amplitude of detection of the (n_1x, n_2y) harmonic.

Finally, we have the multimodal PLL shown in Fig. 6.14.

Figure 6.13 *Diagram of a multi-modal mixer.*

Reprinted with the permission of Cambridge University Press.

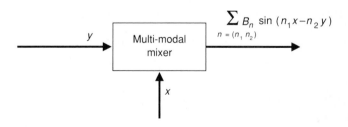

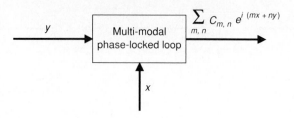

Figure 6.14 *Diagram of a multi-modal PLL.*

We have already seen that the output of the SYN circuit is periodic in each of its inputs, $V(x)$ (from within the cell) and $V(Y)_+$ (forcing the VCON through SYN). Therefore, it can be expanded in a Fourier series thus:

$$P(V(x) + V(y)_+) = \sum_{m,n=-\infty}^{m,n=+\infty} C_{m,n} e^{imx+iny}.$$

SYN is a multimodal mixer, and the VCON circuit (whose schematic has been shown earlier) is a multimodal phase-locked loop.

Hoppensteadt has described the rotation vector method of studying phase locking between timers. This is summarized below not only for completeness, but also because it clarifies the concept of phase locking. Consider,

$$\frac{dx}{dt} = \omega + \varepsilon f(x, \varepsilon),$$

where

$$x = (x_1, \ldots, x_n),$$

f is periodic in each of the components of x, and
ε is small and positive.

If we perform a simple change of variables such that $v = \omega \cdot x$ and $u_j = W_j \cdot x$, then

$$\frac{dv}{dt} = \omega \cdot \frac{dx}{dt},$$

$$\Rightarrow \frac{dv}{dt} = \omega^2 + \varepsilon\omega f(x, \varepsilon),$$

$$\frac{du_j}{dt} = W_j \cdot \frac{dx}{dt},$$

and

$$\Rightarrow \frac{du_j}{dt} = \varepsilon W_j f(x, \varepsilon),$$

if we choose vectors $W_2, \ldots, W_N$ all orthogonal to ω and all pairwise orthogonal.

Note that v is a time-like variable (varying as $\omega^2 t$) and that the variables u_j vary slowly with respect to t. Hoppensteadt then uses the Bogoliuboff's averaging method (whose discussion is beyond the scope of this text) to average the u equations with respect to the time-like variable v.

$$\frac{dU_j}{dt} = \varepsilon W_j \cdot f^*(U_2, \ldots, U_N).$$

It turns out that if the averaged equations for U have an exponentially stable equilibrium (i.e., U tends to U^* as t tends to infinity), then the u components of the original system remain bounded for all time if ε is small.

Now, if we know v and u_j, we can find x:

$$x = v\omega\omega^2 + \sum_{j=2}^{j=N} u_j \frac{W_j}{W_j^2}$$

$$\frac{x}{v} = \frac{\omega}{\omega^2} + \sum_{j=2}^{j=N} u_j \frac{W_j}{W_j^2 v},$$

and since the components of u are bounded,

$$\lim_{t \to \infty} \frac{x}{v} = \frac{\omega}{\omega^2},$$

or

$$x_1 : x_2 : \cdots : x_N \to \omega_1 : \omega_2 : \cdots : \omega_N \qquad \text{as } t \to \infty.$$

ω is the rotation vector because the relative ratios of its components give the relative frequencies of the various clock phases.

Phase locking can now be explained in terms of what has just been presented. Under the conditions just mentioned, it is possible to perturb the free frequencies up to order $O(\varepsilon)$, provided ε remains small, and still have the same limiting ratios. The system is said to be phase locked to the free frequencies. Thus, the rotation vector method demonstrates that a collection of phase-locked clocks behave like a single clock on one time scale having multiple outputs.

If one thinks of the brain as an energy surface, then the valleys would correspond to stable, repeatable brain responses. An external stimulus would set the initial conditions and the brain's firing pattern would dynamically evolve to one of the patterns represented by a valley floor. To construct a mechanical analogue to this sequence of events, the arrival of the external stimulus is akin to placing a ball on an uneven surface and the evolution of the brain's firing pattern is akin to the ball moving on the surface to a position where it has minimal potential energy. The valley floors in the brain model are remembered responses, which may take the form of information recall or behavior modification.

Hoppensteadt's approach suggests that we can discover a frequency-response surface whose valleys represent stable phase-locked combinations of firings. Each neuron has a rich combination of such stable responses, and various connections between neurons can excite various combinations of stable responses.

■ 6.4 Some General Comments on Relaxation Searches

Hopfield networks use relaxation techniques to perform multiple-constraint satisfying searches (i.e., the units in the network iteratively converge to a stable state that represents a "good solution" to the problem). Hinton (1986b) summarizes the questions that must be answered with regard to relaxation searches before they can be applied extensively.

1. Will the network settle down or will it oscillate aimlessly? If it does settle down, how long does this process take?

2. What does the network compute in the process of settling down?

3. How much information does each unit need to convey to its neighbors during the settling-down process?

4. How are the weights that encode the knowledge acquired?

While this book deals primarily with the last of these questions, it is good to reflect on the other questions within whose constraints the present extensive scientific inquiry must proceed. A few general comments regarding relaxation searches deserve mention here. First, with regard to Questions 1 and 2. If a cost can be assigned to each state of the network and if it can be shown that this cost is being minimized at every iteration, then we can be sure that the network is indeed computing something (i.e., it is computing the optimal/minimal-cost state of the network) and that it will stop when this computation is complete. We have already encountered this cost-minimization idea earlier in this chapter. If a linear programming approach is to be taken to this cost minimization, then it should be remembered that there is a very clear-cut distinction between constraints and costs; the former must be satisfied. Therefore, a very low cost solution that violates, say, just one of many constraints is simply inadmissible. But in systems where we wish to apply relaxation networks (e.g., vision systems), we would be willing to accept interpretations that violate a constraint if they satisfy several others. This suggests that the constraints that we require are "weaker." Our constraints have associated plausibilities and the solution we seek is the one that fits these plausible constraints as well as possible (this encompasses the dual considerations of satisfying as many constraints as possible while minimizing cost simultaneously).

Strict enforcement of constraints is implemented by the use of feedback loops (the amount by which the current values violate the constraint is measured and the values are altered to reduce this violation). We can eliminate the separate feedback loops for the constraints and encode the weak constraints directly in the excitatory and inhibitory interconnections. We have allowed for the partial satisfaction of constraints; however, to prevent the network from hedging its bets by settling into a state where many units are slightly active, and to speed up convergence of the network, we use a nonlinear decision rule. Since the output to which the network relaxes is very dependent on the initial state, this suggests that the problem should be encoded in the initial state. The principles of content-addressable memory are apparent here. If the minima represent memory items and if the initial state is a query that represents a position in the space over which the function (which we are minimizing) is defined, then the relaxation is toward the memory item/minima that is closest.

It is possible, in hard problems, for gradient descent to get stuck in local minima as opposed to global minima. There are two alternatives to dealing with this problem. One is to use the problem to create a content-addressable memory as in the Hopfield net, where the local minimum is what is being sought. The other alternative is to determine rules that permit escape from situations where the search is stuck in a local minimum. If we think of the function that we are minimizing as an energy function, then this latter method basically entails occasionally abandoning the continual descent toward lower energy states and jumping to a higher energy state. A simple physical analogy might help to clarify this approach.

Consider the situation where a ball positioned randomly along the landscape is initially equally likely to end up in either A or B. If the system is slightly agitated, there is a greater likelihood of the ball moving from A to B than vice versa. If, on the other hand, the system is vigorously agitated, the likelihood of the ball moving from B to A is just as great as that of moving from A to B. Now, imagine that A is a local minimum that we want to avoid and B is the global minimum that we seek. Then the best strategy would be to start with a vigorous shaking and then gradually slow down the shaking. This technique is akin to the annealing of a metal (wherein a very low energy state of the metal is found by melting it and then slowly reducing the temperature) and is called *simulated annealing* (see Fig. 6.15).

Simulated annealing could be applied to Hopfield nets in the following manner. If the energy gap between the 1 and 0 states of the kth unit in the network is ΔE_k, then regardless of the previous state set, $s_k = 1$ (where s_k is the state of the kth unit) with probability

$$p_k = \frac{1}{(1 + e^{-\Delta E_k/T})},$$

where T is a parameter that acts like system temperature. It turns out that in thermal equilibrium, the relative probability of being in two global states has a Boltzmann distribution

$$\frac{P_\alpha}{P_\beta} = e^{-(E_\alpha - E_\beta)/T},$$

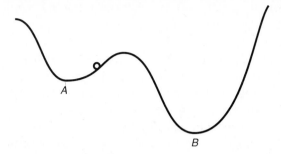

Figure 6.15 *Principle of simulated annealing.*

where P_i is the probability of being in the ith global state and E_i is that state's energy.

The probabilities of the global states are therefore determined by their energy levels. Even though modification of a single weight affects the energies of more than one global state, there is a convenient relation given by Hinton (1986b) that shows the effect of a weight change on each global state. If the visible units are the ones used to specify the patterns to be learned, then

$$\frac{\delta \ln P_\alpha^-}{\delta w_{ij}} = \frac{1}{T}\left[s_i^\alpha s_j^\alpha - \sum_\beta P_\beta^- s_i^\beta s_j^\beta \right],$$

where

> s_i^α = binary state of the ith unit in the αth global state and
> P_α^- = probability, at equilibrium, of global state α of network when no visible unit is constrained to a particular value.

Therefore, the effect of a weight change can be computed from local information relevant only to the nodes that the weight connects. Though this means that global-state probabilities can be easily manipulated if they are known, the fact is that these probabilities are often unknown and it is the task of the network to figure out how to use its hidden units to simulate the behavior of its visible units. Recall that the Widrow-Hoff rule (see Chapter 4) and the perceptron convergence procedure (Chapter 3) failed to solve the XOR problem. That is because these rules were not designed to capture anything beyond second-order structure. Statistically, the separate probability of each visible unit being active captures first-order structure while the $v^2/2$ pairwise correlations (among the v visible units) captures second-order structure. Dealing with higher-order statistics requires the use of more than just the visible units. In order to make it possible to use pairwise connections between units to capture higher-order statistics, we need to express this higher-order structure in terms of the second-order structure of a larger set of units. These extra units are what we have been referring to as the hidden units. Hinton (1986b) refers to the task of learning how to use the extra units as hard learning and points out that the Widrow-Hoff rule is incapable of hard learning. The ability to use local information, at equilibrium, to determine global quantities shows up again in the Boltzmann machine learning algorithm discussed in the next section.

■ 6.5 The Boltzmann Machine Learning Algorithm

If the environment clamps a vector over the visible units and allows the network to attain equilibrium, the complete structure of the environmental ensemble can be given by the probability distribution $P^+(V_a)$ of each of the 2^v vectors over the v visible units. Hinton (1986b) points out that the interpretation of this clamped vector amounts to the network reaching an equilibrium state with this vector as a boundary condition. This distribution is independent of the weights. In contrast, if none of the units are clamped, owing to the stochastic behavior of the units, the network goes through several states and generates its own probability distribution $P^-(V_a)$. A particular set of weights constitutes a perfect model of the environmental structure if it leads to exactly the same probability distribution of visible vectors when the network is running freely with no units being clamped by the environment. An information-theoretic measure of the distance between the environmental and free-running probability distributions is given by

$$G = \sum_\alpha P^+(V_a) \ln \frac{P^+(V_a)}{P^-(V_a)}.$$

This gives the distance in bits from the free-running distribution to the environmental distribution and is sometimes referred to as the asymmetric divergence or the information gain. Minimizing G appears, as above, to be a difficult computational problem given the fact that changing a weight affects the probabilities of many global minima. Again, all the information that is required about the other weights in order to change w_{ij}

appropriately shows up in the behavior of the ith and jth units at thermal equilibrium. The change is given by

$$\frac{\delta G}{\delta w_{ij}} = -\frac{1}{T}[p_{ij}^+ - p_{ij}^-],$$

where

p_{ij}^+ = probability that the ith and jth units are both on when the network is environment driven and

p_{ij}^- = probability that the ith and jth units are both on when the network is free running.

The hidden units have no way of determining whether the information that they receive is an effect of the environmental ambience or simply results from other weights. There is the unwelcome possibility of each part of the network constructing a model of the other and, in the process, ignoring the external environment. The free running of the network acts as a control run. Because of the way in which equilibrium mathematics works it is possible to subtract off the purely internal contribution and use the difference to update the weights.

Determination of the partial derivative of G does not complete the learning algorithm in and of itself. Hinton (1986b) points out that the amount of each weight change has yet to be determined. Also unclear are the solutions to questions such as how long is it necessary to observe statistics before weight change, how many weights should be changed, and the like. While trial and error suffices for simple networks, complications can arise in more complex situations. For example, there is nothing to prevent the creation of very large weights that would result in very large energy barriers that prevent the reaching of equilibrium. Then, the relation used to determine the partial derivative of G no longer holds. To prevent this the weights should be kept small by, for example, the use of weight decay (with the speed of this decay being proportional to the weight's absolute magnitude). The magnitude of a weight now shows how important it is for modeling the environmental structure. There are some side effects though. With small weights, it is no longer possible to make the probability ratios for similar global states very different. This implies that environments where similar vectors have different probabilities will not be modeled well.

■ *6.6 Literature Overview*

Hopfield (1986) lays out the conceptual framework needed to comprehend computation in model neural circuits. This paper provides a succinct explanation of the link between the Hopfield nets and their relation to biology. Hopfield (1985) provides details of the electronic implementation of the Hopfield net and discusses the traveling salesman problem at some length. Simulation results and variants of the TSP are also discussed. Hopfield (1984) demonstrates that neurons with graded response have collective computational properties akin to those of two-state neurons. Much of the material in Section 6.2 is derived from these sources and the reader is encouraged to consult them for detail.

Section 6.2.5 gives a brief introduction to some recent work done by Platt (1987) on constrained differential optimization. This paper is a good source for a discussion of some of the classical methods of constrained optimization. This chapter has discussed BDMM (basic differential multiplier method) in a very introductory fashion. That discussion was motivated by the application of BDMM to the traveling salesman problem. Much greater detail on BDMM can be found in the source. In particular, the paper discusses the application of BDMM to another neural problem — analog decoding.

Takeda (1986) provides a discussion of the material in Sections 6.2.7, 6.2.8, and 6.2.9. The paper may be consulted for the application of the number representation schemes mentioned in this chapter to the Hitchcock problem (a "flow" problem that finds a flow that finds a minimum cost solution to the problem of satisfying a certain number of demands from a certain number of sources). There is also a discussion of the solution of simultaneous equations on a neural network.

Section 6.3 is a distillation of some of the interesting ideas from Hoppensteadt's (1986) book. This source provides a wealth of detail regarding the material presented in this chapter and on other relevant material beyond the scope of this book.

Hinton (1986b) provided the material for Sections 6.4 and 6.5. This source offers a derivation of the Boltzmann machine learning algorithm and an example of hard learning.

Activation: The state of a particular processing unit at a particular time. Especially in a model not using distributed representation of information, the degree of activation could indicate the degree of confidence that a particular feature is present or absent, rather than providing merely a yes/no answer concerning the presence or absence of a particular feature. Alternatively, the degree of activation could suggest the quantity of a feature that is present.

Adaptation: The process by which much of learning proceeds in a neural network. Adaptation is relatively easily done in a system using distributed processing.

Adaptive Network: An adaptive system, having relatively simple units, that functions in a decentralized, highly parallel manner.

Adaptive Resonance Theory: A variety of learning strategy that attempts to eliminate some of the temporal instabilities of competitive learning by embedding a competitive learning model into a self-regulating structure whose autonomous learning and recognition proceed stably in response to an arbitrary input pattern sequence.

Adaptive System: In its most general form, one that modifies its structure as a function of its experience in order to improve relative to some criterion.

Association Model: A connectionist neuronal model based on the tenet that repetitive activation of a synapse, when it contributes to the firing of a recipient neuron, increases the effectiveness of the synapse—used to study adaptive networks. (*See* Reinforcement Model.)

Associative Memory: One that hinges on the ability to get from one internal representation to another or to infer a complex representation from a portion of it. In conventional memory systems, on the other hand, a particular item must be accessed by providing its unique memory address.

Associative Recall: The retrieval of information based on the association of its representative activity pattern with the activity pattern supplied as the "key" or "memory address." (*See also* Associative Memory and Content Addressable Memory.)

Automatic Programming: *See* Learning.

Back-Propagation Paradigm: *See* Generalized Delta Rule.

Basic Differential Multiplier Method (BDMM): Proposed by Platt (1987), an alternative to differential gradient descent used to estimate Lagrange multiples.

Boltzmann Machine: A learning model that develops a learning procedure capable of learning an internal representation.

Capacity Catastrophe: A problem that occurs in non–self-stablizing systems when an unlimited input stream causes memories of prior learning to be washed away.

Cognitron: A multilayered neural network that employs competitive learning. It was developed by Fukushima (1975) in response to the observation that the neural nets in the visual centers of the brain developed so as to recognize features in the input patterns presented to them.

Competitive Learning: An essentially nonassociative statistical scheme that employs simple, unsupervised learning rules so that useful hidden units develop.

Complete Correlation Matrix Memory (CCMM): One that has connections for all possible pairs (i, j) and only one of a type.

Computational Complexity: Roughly speaking, the number of steps that an algorithm takes to get an answer—a measure that is more appropriate in von Neumann computers than in neural networks. (*See* Von Neumann Machines and Programming Complexity.)

Connectable Area: The region from which a cell can have its afferent (input) synapses.

Connectionism: Very broadly, an approach to computing born out of the hypothesis that the complex structure needed for problem solving might be encoded in the neuronal interconnection pattern. Growing out of a marriage between the principles of continuous and symbolic systems, connectionism is a concept basic to some of the developments in neural networks.

Constrained Differential Optimization: Generally a problem that can be expressed as minimize $f(x)$ subject to $g(x) = 0$, where x is the state of the network. x should evolve such that it is attracted to the constraining subspace ($g(x) = 0$) and then glides along it until it finds the locally smallest occurrence of f.

Content Addressable Memory: One that provides a portion of the content of an item to be retrieved as the item's memory address. It is clearly linked with the concept of pattern recognition—that is, the pattern created by a portion of the content of an item should be recognized as that created by the entire item.

Control System: A goal-seeking system with non–goal-seeking components (*see* Goal-Seeking System). The human brain is an example of a control system.

Cross-Talk: Interference effects that are one of the fundamental problems associated with holographic memory models. Without orthogonality, cross-talk becomes more severe as the number of associations becomes very large.

Cybernetics: The study of self-organizing machines. Cyberneticians are preoccupied with developing systems that learn.

Delta Rule: A learning strategy typically applied to the case in which pairs of patterns—an input pattern and a target output pattern—are to be associated, where the contents of specific patterns do not matter as much as the pattern of correlations among the patterns. (Also called the Widrow-Hoff Rule and the Least Mean Square Method.)

Depolarization: The neuronal state of heterostatic units that can be equated with pleasure in a biological analogy of information processing.

Deterministic Algorithm: One whose operation is known in advance. (Compare Stochastic Algorithm.)

Distributed Processing: The distribution of processing among several processors.

Distributed Representation: A technique whereby particular concepts or items need not correspond to particular processing elements in neural networks. Sometimes it is more appropriate to represent concepts and other pieces of information by collective states of neural networks. Thus a pattern of activity over several processing elements, rather than the activity of a particular element, represents an item. This collective representation is called an *holographic* or *hologic representation.*

Emergent Properties: These properties represent a particular stage in a sequential thought process in each distributed architecture and cause the model to appear, in hindsight, as if it did indeed "know the rules."

Expert Systems: Those systems having problem solving expertise in a specialized domain. Such systems have two kinds of knowledge—readily available textbook knowledge and often domain-specific heuristics that can be employed to solve problems using that textbook knowledge.

Exponential Time Algorithm: One for which a bound on time complexity cannot be expressed in the manner that it can for polynomial time algorithms. (*See* Polynomial Time Algorithm.)

Feedforward Network: One in which every processing unit in any layer must get inputs from layers lower than its own and must send outputs to layers higher than its own (where lower layers are defined as those closer to the input layer and higher layers are defined as those closer to the output layer). This property allows the output vector to be computed by a forward pass that computes the activity of each layer in turn using the already computed activity levels in earlier layers.

Forced Learning: Refers to the intermediate continuum of rules based on the manipulation of the content of the input stimulus stream to bring about learning. (Compare Competitive and Spontaneous Learning.)

Fuzzy Sets: Classes of objects in which the transition from membership to nonmembership is gradual rather than abrupt.

Generalized Delta Rule: An extension to the delta rule wherein learning proceeds by back-propagation of error signals. (*See* Delta Rule.)

Goal-Seeking System: One that utilizes feedback information to move toward, or to maintain, a particular system state that is the predetermined goal.

Gradient Descent: The technique used to approach a minimal solution in a mathematically defined space by progressively moving in the direction of steepest descent (at each iteration of a multiple step process, the move is in the direction of steepest descent at the current position in space).

Hebbian Rule: A learning strategy, due to D. O. Hebb, that suggests that when a cell *A* repeatedly and persistently participates in firing cell *B*, then *A*'s efficiency in firing *B* is increased.

Heterostasis: The condition toward which the somatic nervous system moves as it strives to maximize the difference between the amounts of received rewards and punishments. Intelligence in complex systems can be thought of as a concomitant of striving to maximize heterostasis.

Heterostat: A connectionist neural model of the generalized reinforcement type developed by Klopf (1982) in response to his perception of the similarities between social and neural systems.

Holographic (Hologic) Representation: *See* Distributed Representation.

Homeostasis: A term borrowed from biology that refers to the ability of higher animals to maintain an internal constancy (e.g., body temperature) regardless of external conditions. (Compare Heterostasis.)

Hyperplanar Separability: The property that a collection of points in space is said to possess if a hyperplane can be found that separates them into at least two nonoverlapping sets. In two dimensions, a set of points is linearly separable if a line can be found that divides the set into two nonoverlapping sets.

Hyperpolarization: The neuronal state of heterostatic units that can be equated with pain in a biological analogy of information processing.

Incomplete Correlation Matrix Memory (ICMM): One in which pairs are selected or generated randomly.

Information-Processing Models: Memory models that conceive of man as an information-processing system executing internal programs for testing, comparing, analyzing, manipulating, and storing information.

Informax Principle: Concept whereby, at least in an intuitive way,

a Hebbian rule may act to generate a cell whose output activity preserves maximum information about the input activities.

Interactive Activation Model: Proposed as capable of explaining the fundamental facts of word perception, a model in which interlevel connections are selectively excitatory or inhibititory.

Interconnection Pattern: In connectionist models, that which forms the analogue to algorithms in conventional computers.

Lateral Inhibition: Mutually inhibitory connections between elements in, say, a PDP model, representing mutually incompatible concepts. See examples of competitive learning in the text.

Learning: The process accomplished by incorporating past experience into interconnection patterns in neural nets. Also called Automatic Programming.

Learning Machine: One that profits from its experience. The perceptron is an example.

Learning Rule: The strategy employed to alter the weights (*see* Weights) in a neural net whenever the net learns something in response to new inputs or to changes in the environment.

Least Mean Square Method: *See* Delta Rule.

Locality: The notion of a single processor (e.g., in a PDP model) depending only on the processors in its vicinity for its data and communication needs. Locality permits modularity in construction of the model and allows for relatively easy adaptability to external change by, for example, making possible replacement of a single processor with largely local changes in processor linkages.

McCulloch–Pitts Neurons: In early theoretical studies, biological neurons modeled as logical decision elements described by a two-valued state variable and organized into logical decision networks that could compute Boolean functions. The model failed, however, to capture analog processing and high interconnectivity, both important aspects of biological neurons.

Minimal Energy Concept: The theory whereby, in neural networks, energy is a global quantity not felt by the individual processing unit. Stable-state configurations of the net correspond to local energy minima and, as a neural net computes the solution to a problem, the configuration evolves to one of the minima.

Momentary Stimulus Perceptron: A perceptron with no capability for pattern recognition.

Multilayered Perceptron: A perceptron having one or more layers separating the input and output layers.

Neocognitron: An augmented hierarchical model designed to resolve the cognitron's primary flaw—that its response was severely affected by a shift in position of and/or by a distortion in the shape of input patterns, which limited its use as a pattern recognition device.

Nondeterministic Algorithm: One that is best viewed as having two stages—guessing and checking. The first stage involves guessing the solution to a problem; the second stage is checking to see whether the solution is appropriate.

Non–Goal-Seeking System: Essentially an open-loop system. (Compare Goal-Seeking System.)

Nonrecurrent Network: *See* Feedforward Network.

NP: A class of problems for which a nondeterministic algorithm exists that solves the problem in polynomial time.

NP-**Complete:** A class of problems such that for a particular *NP*-complete problem every instance of every problem in *NP* can be converted to an instance of this particular problem, and this conversion can be affected in polynomial time.

Orthogonal Learning: Learning in which nonorthogonal patterns are orthogonalized by a network of neuron-like elements relying on the Widrow-Hoff rule.

P: A class of problems such that if a problem is in *P* there exists a deterministic algorithm that solves it in polynomial time.

Parallel Distributed Processing (PDP) Models: Ones comprised of a large number of simple processing elements interacting with others via excitatory and inhibitory connections. PDP models are used extensively in the study of neural nets.

Perceptron: A neural net that undergoes supervised training and is used as an associative memory. In the words of Rosenblatt (*Principles of Neurodynamics*, 1962), perceptrons are "simplified networks designed to permit the study of lawful relationships between the organization of a nerve net, the organization of its environment, and the 'psychological' performances of which it is capable."

Phase Locking: A phenomenon that explains how large, complicated networks can synchronize in stable ways.

Phase-Locked Loops: Basic parts of electronic timing circuits that are based on the phenomenon of phase locking.

Photo-Perceptron: A perceptron that treats optical signals as stimuli.

Physical System Models: Memory models that seek a way to utilize an interconnected collection of relatively simple elements to implement the basic functions of associative memory. (Compare Information Processing Models.)

Plastic System: *See* Adaptive System.

Polynomial Time Algorithm: One that operates in polynomial time if its time complexity function is $O(p(n))$, where p is some polynomial function of input size n.

Principal Component Analysis: A method for identifying interesting but unanticipated structure (e.g., clustering) in high-dimensional data sets.

Principle of Incompatibility: A theory stating that, as the complexity of a system increases, our ability to make precise and significant statements about its behavior diminishes until a threshold is reached beyond which precision and significance — or relevance — become almost mutually exclusive characteristics. As it relates to cognition and neural networks, the basis for the fuzzy set theories depends on this principle.

Principle of Virtual Images: A theory that basically states that there is a component to the new output that is attributable to memory recollections. This principle explains the changes in output that result from modifications in the network.

Programming Complexity: A measure best described by the number of arithmetic operations that must be performed to determine the proper interconnection strengths and neural biases for a problem's solution. In a von Neumann computer, a program once written can act on several sets of data. Since data and instructions are not separable in a neural network, the interconnections and biases must be altered for each new data set. Programming complexity is often a more appropriate measure of complexity for neural networks than computational complexity.

Reading: In an adaptive filter model, the transformation of the input signals in a network.

Reinforcement Model: A connectionist neural model in which sequential rather than simultaneous events are of fundamental importance and in which an instrumental conditioning orientation is adopted.

Relaxation Property: In a network, the network's method of iteratively approaching the best solution to the problem.

Spontaneous Learning: A type that proceeds by completely unsupervised discovery. (Compare Competitive Learning and Forced Learning.)

Standard Regularization Theory: A technique which solves problems in terms of quadratic energy functionals that must be minimized.

Statistical Models: Systems that, when faced with a classification problem, serially compute the most likely classification, and in which parameters are derived from training data. Neural nets, on the other hand, compute parallel and use those computations to adjust internal interconnection patterns.

Stimulus Substitution: Procedure by which, if stimulus A elicits response R_A, and if stimulus B is usually associated with A, then B will eventually elicit response R_A. A has been substituted for *B*. This is what Hebb's rule essentially states. (*See* Hebbian Rule.)

Stochastic Algorithm: A probabilistic algorithm.

Supervised Strategy: In the training of a neural net, the technique that specifies the correct class for an input pattern during the presentation of that input pattern. Nets trained under supervision are used as associative memories. (Compare Unsupervised Learning.)

Symmetry: Property that occurs in neural nets when the synaptic strength and sign (i.e., the weight on the interconnection) of the interconnection from neuron *i* to neuron *j* is the same as on the interconnection from neuron *j* to neuron *i*. (*See* Weight.)

Teacher: In supervised learning, the device, procedure, or method that accomplishes network conditioning, often by error correction.

Two-Thirds Rule: A concept in adaptive resonance theory models that is used to permit subliminal sensitizing of the network in preparation for an example of an expected class of input patterns.

Unsupervised Learning: Strategy in which the correct class for an input pattern is not specified when the input pattern is presented. Nets trained in this manner are used as vector quantizers or to form clusters. (Compare Supervised Learning.)

Vicinity Area: The region to which a cell's efferent (output) synapses connect.

Von Neumann Machine: Name given to conventional computer systems wherein there is a clear distinction between the central processor and the memory system. The von Neumann bottleneck refers to the limitation in attainable processing speed because of the bottleneck caused by the need for communication between these two distinct components. To use programs and data stored in memory, it is necessary that relevant information be directed through the sequential processor.

Voltage Controlled Ocillator Neuron (VCON): An electrical model, made possible by integrated circuitry, that is specifically designed to facilitate the study of neuronal frequency-response properties.

Weights: Property that refers to the characterization of inter-unit interconnections (whose biological analog is a synapse). The characterization has two features—its nature (i.e., whether it is excitatory or inhibitory) and the degree of influence that the unit from which the interconnection begins has on the incident unit.

Widrow-Hoff Rule: *See* Delta Rule.

Writing: In an adaptive filter model, writing comes about when each input pattern produces adaptive changes in the neuronal interconnections.

Bibliography

Arbib (1975): Arbib, M. A., From Automata Theory to Brain Theory, *International Journal of Man-Machine Studies* 7: 279–295.

Baum (1988): Baum, E. B., On the Capabilities of Multilayer Perceptrons, *Journal of Complexity*, 4: 193–215.

Baum (1989): Baum, E. B., and Haussler, D., What Size Net Gives Valid Generalization?, to appear in *Neural Computation*.

Blumer (1989): Blumer, A., Ehrenfeucht, A., Haussler, D., and Warmuth, M., Learnability and the Vapnik–Chervonenkis Dimension, to appear in *Journal of Association of Computing Machinery*.

Carpenter (1988): Carpenter, G., and Grossberg, S., The ART of Adaptive Pattern Recognition by a Self-Organizing Neural Network, *Computer*, (March) 77–87.

Chandrasekaran (1981): Chandrasekaran, B., Natural and Social System Metaphors for Distributed Problem Solving: Introduction to the Issue, *IEEE Transactions of Systems, Man, and Cybernetics* SMC-11, no. 1 (January): 1–5.

Cybenko (1989): Cybenko, G., Approximation by Superpositions of a Sigmoidal Function, to appear in *Mathematic Control Systems Signals*, 2.

Duda (1973): Duda, R., and Hart, P., *Pattern Classification and Scene Analysis*, Wiley–Interscience Series.

Dutta (1988): Dutta, S., and Shekhar, S., Bond Rating: A Non-Conservative Application of Neural Networks, *IEEE International Conference on Neural Networks*, San Diego, CA, July 24–27, II: 443–450.

Eichmann (1985): Eichmann, G., and Caulfield, H. J., Optical Learning (Inference) Machines, *Applied Optics* 24, no. 14 (July): 2051–2054.

Farhat (1985): Farhat, N., and Psaltis, D., Prata, A., and Paek, E., Optical Implementation of the Hopfield Model, *Applied Optics* 24, no. 10, (May): 1459–1475.

Feldman (1988): Feldman, J., Fanty, M., and Goddard, N., Computing with Structured Neural Networks, *Computer,* (March): 91–103.

Fukushima (1975): Fukushima, K., Cognitron: A Self-Organizing Multilayered Neural Network, *Biological Cybernetics* 20: 121–136.

Fukushima (1980): Fukushima, K., Neocognitron: A Self-Organizing Neural Network Model for a Mechanism of Pattern Recognition Unaffected by Shift in Position, *Biological Cybernetics* 36: 193–202.

Fukushima (1986): Fukushima, K., A Neural Network Model for Selective Attention in Visual Pattern Recognition, *Biological Cybernetics* 55: 5–15.

Fukushima (1988): Fukushima, K., A Neural Network for Visual Pattern Recognition, *Computer* (March): 65–75.

Gallant (1988): Gallant, S. I., Connectionist Expert Systems, *Communications of the ACM* 31, no. 2 (February): 152–169.

Garey (1979): Garey, M. R., and Johnson, D. S., *Computers and Intractability: A Guide to the Theory of NP-Completeness,* San Francisco: W. H. Freeman & Co.

Gray (1988): Gray, D. L., Michek, A. N., and Porod, W., *Application of Neural Networks to Sorting Problems,* Department of Electrical & Computer Engineering, Notre Dame, IN: University of Notre Dame.

Grossberg (1976): Grossberg, S., Adaptive Pattern Classification and Universal Recoding: II. Feedback, Expectation, Olfaction, Illusions, *Biological Cybernetics* 23: 187–202.

Grossberg (1987a): Grossberg, S., Competitive Learning: From Interactive Activation to Adaptive Resonance, *Cognitive Science* 11: 23–63.

Grossberg (1987b): Grossberg, S. [Ed.], *The Adaptive Brain,* New York: North-Holland Publishers.

Hartigan (1975): Hartigan, J., *Clustering Algorithms,* Wiley Series in Probability and Mathematical Statistics, New York: John Wiley & Sons.

Hebb (1949): Hebb, D.O., *The Organization of Behavior, A Neuropsychological Theory,* New York: John Wiley & Sons.

Hinton (1981): Hinton, G., and Anderson, J. [Eds.], *Parallel Models of Associative Memory,* Lawrence Erlbaum Associates, Publishers.

Hinton (1986a): Hinton, G., McClelland, J. L., and Rumelhart, D. E., Distributed Representations, Chapter 3 in *Parallel Distributed Processing, Explorations in the Microstructure of Cognition, Vol. 1: Foundations* [Eds.: Rumelhart, D., and McClelland, J., and the PDP Research Group], Cambridge, MA: The MIT Press.

Hinton (1986b): Hinton, G., and Sejnowski, T., Learning and Relearning in Boltzmann Machines, Chapter 7 in *Parallel Distributed Processing, Explorations in the Microstructure of Cognition, Vol. 1: Foundations* [Eds.: Rumelhart, D., and McClelland, J., and the PDP Research Group], Cambridge, MA: The MIT Press.

Hopfield (1984): Hopfield, J., Neurons with Graded Response Have Collective Computational Properties Like Those of Two-State Neurons, *Proceedings of the National Academy of Science USA* 81, (May) 3088–3092.

Hopfield (1985): Hopfield, J., and Tank, D., "Neural" Computation of Decisions in Optimization Problems, *Biological Cybernetics* 52: 141–152.

Hopfield (1986): Hopfield, J., and Tank, D., Computing with Neural Circuits: A Model, *Science* 233: 625–633.

Hoppensteadt (1986): Hoppensteadt, F. C., *An Introduction to the Mathematics of Neurons,* New York: Cambridge University Press.

Judd (1987): Judd, S., Learning in Networks is Hard, IEEE First International Conference on Neural Networks, San Diego, CA, June 21–24, II: 685–692.

Klimasauskas (1987): Klimasauskas, C.C., *The 1987 Annotated Neuro Computing Bibliography,* Servichley, PA: Neuroconnection.

Klopf (1982): Klopf, A. H., *The Hedonistic Neuron: A Theory of Memory, Learning and Intelligence,* New York: Hemisphere Publishing Corporation.

Koch (1986): Koch, C., Marroquin, J., and Yuille, A., Analog "Neuronal" Networks in Early Vision, *Proceedings of the National Academy of Sciences, USA* 83 (June): 4263–4267.

Kohonen (1972): Kohonen, T., Correlation Matrix Memories, *IEEE Transactions on Computers* C-21, no. 4 (April): 353–359.

Kohonen (1977): Kohonen, T., Lehtio, P., Rovamo, J., Hyvarinen, J., Bry, K., and Vainio, L., A Principle of Neural Associative Memory, *Neuroscience* 2: 1065–1076.

Kohonen (1979): Kohonen, T., *Content-Addressable Memories,* Springer Series in Information Sciences 1.

Kohonen (1981): Kohonen, T., Lehtio, P., Oja, 'Distributed Associative Memory,' Chapter 4 in *Parallel Models of Associative Memory,* [Eds.: Hinton, G., and Anderson, J.], Lawrence Erlbaum Associates, Publishers.

Kohonen (1983): Kohonen, T., *Self-Organization and Associative Memory,* Springer Series in Information Sciences 8.

Linsker (1986): Linsker, R., From Basic Network Principles to Neural Architecture (series), *Proceedings of the National Academy of Sciences USA* 83 (October–November): 7508–7512, 8390–8394, 8779–8783.

Linsker (1988): Linsker, R., Self-Organization in a Perceptual Network, *Computer* (March): 105–117.

Lippmann (1987): Lippmann, R., An Introduction to Computing with Neural Nets, *IEEE ASSP Magazine* (April): 4–22.

Mada (1985): Mada, H., Architecture for Optical Computing Using Holographic Associative Memories, *Applied Optics* 24, no. 14 (July): 2063–2066.

McClelland (1981): McClelland, J., and Rumelhart, D., An Interactive Activation Model of Context Effects in Letter Perception: Part 1. An Account of Basic Findings, *Psychological Review* 88, no. 5: 375–407.

McClelland (1986): McClelland, J. L., Rumelhart, D. E., and Hinton, G. E., The Appeal of Parallel Distributed Processing, Chapter 1 in *Parallel Distributed Processing, Explorations in the Microstructure of Cognition, Vol. 1: Foundations* [Eds.: Rumelhart, D., McClelland, J., and the PDP Research Group].

McCulloch (1943): McCulloch, W. S., and Pitts, W. H.: 'A Logical Calculus of the Ideas Immanent in Nervous Activity', Bulletin of Mathematical Biophysics 5: 115–133.

Minsky (1969): Minsky, M., and Papert, S., *Perceptrons: An Introduction to Computational Geometry*, Cambridge, MA: The MIT Press.

Nakano (1972): Nakano, K., Associatron—A Model of Associative Memory, *IEEE Transactions on Systems, Man, and Cybernetics* SMC-2, no. 3 (July): 380–388.

Newell (1983): Newell, A., 'Intellectual Issues in the History of Artificial Intelligence' in *The Study of Information: Interdisciplinary Messages*, [Eds.: Machlup, F., and Mansfield, U.], New York: John Wiley & Sons.

Noetzel (1988): Noetzel, A. S., and Graziano, M. J., *Comparisons of Sigmoid Functions for Neural Network Convergence*, Department EE/CS, Brooklyn, N.Y.: Polytechnic University and Jericho, N.Y.: Covidea.

Platt (1987): Platt, J. C., and Barr, A. H., *Constrained Differential Optimization*, Pasadena, CA: California Institute of Technology. Preprint to appear in Proceedings of the 1987 IEEE NIPS Conference.

Psaltis (1985): Psaltis, D., and Farhat, N., Optical Information Processing Based on an Associative-Memory Model of Neural Nets with Thresholding and Feedback, *Optics Letters* 10, no. 2 (February): 98–100.

Qian (1988): Qian, N., and Sejnowski, T. J., Predicting the Secondary Structure of Globular Proteins Using Neural Network Models, *Journal of Molecular Biology*, 202: 865–884.

Reicher (1969): Reicher, G. M., Perceptual Recognition as a Function of Meaningfulness of Subject Material, *Journal of Experimental Psychology*, 81: 274–280.

Rosch (1978): Rosch, E., and Lloyd, B. [Eds.], *Cognition and Categorization*, Lawrence Erlbaum Associates, Publishers.

Rosenblatt (1958): Rosenblatt, F., The Perceptron: A Probabilistic Model for Information Storage and Organization in the Brain, *Psychological Review*, 65, no. 6: 386–408.

Rosenblatt (1962): Rosenblatt, F., *Principles of Neurodynamics*, Spartan.

Rumelhart (1982): Rumelhart, D., and McClelland, J., An Interactive Activation Model of Context Effects in Letter Perception: Part 2. The Contextual Enhancement Effect and Extensions of the Model, *Psychological Review* 89, no. 1: 60–94.

Rumelhart (1985): Rumelhart, D., and Zipser, D., Feature Discovery by Competitive Learning, *Cognitive Science* 9: 75–112.

Rumelhart (1986a): Rumelhart, D., Hinton, G., and McClelland, J., A General Framework for Parallel Distributed Processing, Chapter 2 in *Parallel Distributed Processing, Explorations in the Microstructure of Cognition, Vol. 1: Foundations* [Eds.: Rumelhart, D., McClelland, J., and the PDP Research Group], Cambridge, MA: The MIT Press.

Rumelhart (1986b): Rumelhart, D., and McClelland, J., PDP Models and General Issues in Cognitive Science, Chapter 4 in *Parallel Distributed Processing, Explorations in the Microstructure of Cognition, Vol. 1: Foundations* [Eds.: Rumelhart, D., McClelland, J., and the PDP Research Group], Cambridge, MA: The MIT Press.

Rumelhart (1986c): Rumelhart, D., Hinton, G., and Williams, R., Learning Internal Representations by Error Propagation, Chapter 8 in *Parallel Distributed Processing, Explorations in the Microstructure of Cognition, Vol. 1: Foundations* [Eds.: Rumelhart, D., McClelland, J., and the PDP Research Group], Cambridge, MA: The MIT Press.

Sklansky (1973): Sklansky, J., *Pattern Recognition: Introduction and Foundations*, Benchmark Papers in Electrical Engineering and Computer Science, Dowden, Hutchinson & Ross, Inc.

Smolensky (1986): Smolensky, P., Neural and Conceptual Interpretation of PDP Models, Chapter 22 in *Parallel Distributed Processing, Explorations in the Microstructure of Cognition, Vol. 2* [Eds.: Rumelhart, D., McClelland, J., and the PDP Research Group], Cambridge, MA: The MIT Press.

Soon (1988): Soon, V. C., and Huang, Y. F., *Artificial Neural Networks with Second Order Discriminant Functions*, Department of Electrical and Computer Engineering, Notre Dame, IN: University of Notre Dame.

Stent (1973): Stent, G. S., A Physiological Mechanism for Hebbs Postulate of Learning, *Proceedings of the National Academy of Sciences, U.S.A.*, 70, 997–1001.

Stone (1986): Stone, G. O., An Analysis of the Delta Rule and the Learning of Statistical Associations, Chapter 11 in *Parallel Distributed Processing, Explorations in the Microstructure of Cognition, Vol. 1: Foundations* [Eds.: Rumelhart, D., McClelland, J., and the PDP Research Group], Cambridge, MA: The MIT Press.

Sutton (1981): Sutton, R., and Barto, A., Toward a Modern Theory of Adaptive Networks: Expectation and Prediction, *Psychological Review* 88, no. 2: 135–170.

Takeda (1986): Takeda, M., and Goodman, J. W., Neural Networks for Computation: Number Representations and Programming Complexity, *Applied Optics* 25, no. 18 (Septemer): 3033–3046.

Tank (1986): Tank, D., and Hopfield, J., Simple "Neural" Optimization Networks: An A/D Converter, Signal Decision Circuit, and a Linear Programming Circuit, *IEEE Transactions on Circuits and Systems* CAS-33, no. 5, (May): 533–541.

Uttley (1970): Uttley, A. M.: The Informon: A Network for Adaptive Pattern Recognition, *Journal of Theoretical Biology* 27: 31–67.

Valiant (1988): Valiant, L.G., Functionality in Neural Nets, from *Proceedings of AAAI-88*, National Conference on AI. Sponsored by the American Association for Artificial Intelligence.

Williams (1986): Williams, R. J., The Logic of Activation Functions, Chapter 10 in *Parallel Distributed Processing, Explorations in the Microstructure of Cognition, Vol. 1: Foundations* [Eds.: Rumelhart, D., McClelland, J., and the PDP Research Group], Cambridge, MA: The MIT Press.

Zadeh (1973): Zadeh, L., Outline of a New Approach to the Analysis of Complex Systems and Decision Processes, *IEEE Transactions on Systems, Man and Cybernetics* SMC-3, no. 1, (January): 28–44.

 *Index*

Page numbers in *italics* refer to figures; page numbers followed by **t** indicate tabular material.

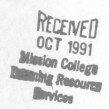